RUNNER'S WORLD

RUN LESS
RUN FASTER

RUNNER'S WORLD

RUN LESS
RUN FASTER

BECOME A FASTER, STRONGER RUNNER WITH THE REVOLUTIONARY 3-RUNS-A-WEEK TRAINING PROGRAM

From the Experts at FIRST℠
BILL PIERCE, SCOTT MURR, and RAY MOSS

FOREWORD BY AMBY BURFOOT, BOSTON MARATHON WINNER

RODALE.

Revised Direct online and Trade paperback editions are being published simultaneously in 2012.

Foreword by Amby Burfoot

Rodale books may be purchased for business or promotional use or for special sales. For information, please write to:
Special Markets Department, Rodale Inc., 733 Third Avenue, New York, NY 10017

Runner's World is a registered trademark of Rodale Inc.

Printed in the United States of America
Rodale Inc. makes every effort to use acid-free ⊗, recycled paper ♲.

Photographs by Mitch Mandel
Book design by Christopher Rhoads

Library of Congress Cataloging-in-Publication Data is on file with the publisher.

ISBN 978–1–60961–802–5 trade paperback
ISBN 978–1–60961–914–5 direct hardcover

Distributed to the trade by Macmillan

13 15 17 19 20 18 16 14 12   trade paperback
2   4   6   8   10 9   7   5   3   direct hardcover

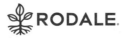

We inspire and enable people to improve their lives and the world around them.
www.rodalebooks.com

CONTENTS

Section IV: Supplemental Training

Section V: Boston and Beyond

FOREWORD

I have long been a fan of the FIRST (Furman Institute of Running and Scientific Training) training program, and the dedicated people who created it (and continue to improve it). Still, after the first edition of *Run Less, Run Faster* was published, I started getting lots of questions from personal and email friends. In addition, I heard similar questions over and over again when I spoke at clinics and runners' expos.

Does the FIRST training program work? How could it, given that it focuses primarily on just three workouts a week? Seems too easy to believe.

We runners are skeptical. We don't believe in free lunches, shoes guaranteed to prevent injuries, or foods that "melt away" the pounds.

We believe in a consistent, disciplined work ethic. We know that's the way to improve. How could the FIRST promise of fewer miles and workouts possibly succeed? Sounds shady.

I found the questions easy to answer. To begin, I told everyone, the FIRST program isn't easy. Just try a few of the workouts—they're tough! Second, many runners fail to reach their running goals because they overtrain—they run too many mediocre workouts and not enough targeted workouts. As a result, they're always tired but haven't necessarily boosted their fitness and their racing potential. That's where the FIRST approach shines.

Happily, I've been able to convince a fair number of runners that less can be more. And almost invariably, the runners who tried the FIRST training program described in *Run Less, Run Faster* reported that it was a great success.

No, I'm not going to exaggerate and say they all set personal records. Many did, but some didn't. However, even those who failed to get faster said they learned much about themselves and the best ways to train by following the program. They often recommended it to friends, which explains why *Run Less, Run Faster* has been one of *Runner's World*'s best-selling books for the past 5 years.

Now here's the new edition. It's got all the great workouts and schedules of the first edition, along with new findings Bill Pierce, Scott Murr, and Ray Moss have gleaned from countless email exchanges with FIRST training program users and from annual running camps they have organized each year at Furman University.

Below is the introduction to *Run Less, Run Faster* that I wrote 5 years ago. I feel even more positive about the program today than I did then, because now it's been road-tested by literally thousands of runners.

Amby Burfoot
Editor-at-Large, Runner's World
June 2011

Given the time-stressed lives that we lead, all runners have the same goal: to run the best we can with the limited amount of time at our disposal. After work, family, daily errands, and keeping up with piles of laundry, how ya gonna fit in enough good workouts to reach your goals? It's the biggest running challenge we face. And Bill Pierce, Scott Murr, and Ray Moss have the answer with the FIRST training program. I know no other training system that comes close to providing the proven, efficient one you'll discover in this book.

But I don't want you to think that the FIRST training program is easy. It isn't. I learned this the hard way a couple of Aprils ago when I visited Bill and his colleagues at Furman University in Greenville, South Carolina, and spent several days training with them. In particular, I ran with Bill and his brother, Don. We learned that we're all about the same age and ability level over a low-fat Italian dinner on my first night in town. The next day, we ran one of Bill's favorite interval workouts, 5 × 1000 meters on a gorgeous curving path along a tree-lined lake on the Furman campus. We warmed up with a relaxed mile or two, and then began the 1000-meter repeats, I thought I was in good shape at the time, but it took all my resolve to match strides with Bill. While I wouldn't say I was running 100 percent, I certainly wasn't lollygagging. Call it a 98 percent effort. I was pooped.

Fortunately, the FIRST method conceived by the team of professors and coaches at the Furman Institute of Running and Scientific Training (FIRST) provides plenty of recovery between hard efforts. I was happy to take the next day off and simply stroll around campus for 30 minutes. Bill played tennis.

That brought us to Day Three, a tempo training day. After another several-mile warmup, Bill and Scott took off on a steady 4-mile run that was supposed to be hard but controlled. For them, I think it was. For me, however, it was too much. I lagged about 30 seconds behind Bill, wondering how he could run hard again just 48 hours after our 1000-meter repeats. The obvious answer: He's been training this way for nearly 20 years. He has adapted to the FIRST program and gotten stronger and faster with it. I hadn't been following the FIRST program . . . though it didn't take me long to decide that I should. Who doesn't want the most fuel-efficient car, or mortgage with the lowest interest rate, or the runners' training program that provides the best results in the least amount of time? I most appreciate that the FIRST approach is scientifically based and meticulously measured. Many coaches and personal trainers develop their plans according to their "proven successes." Unfortunately, they've got no scientific or statistical analysis to back up their claims. They might be good enough coaches, but they've never actually studied how well their plans work.

Bill, Ray, and Scott have—extensively.

The members of the FIRST team were college professors before they became coaches and have always approached the FIRST system as a scientific experiment. They've measured all their runners before and after beginning the FIRST program, and the results could very well have proven the system an absolute bust. But that's not what happened. Instead, the experiments have produced consistently spectacular outcomes. The runners train less than they used to, and 16 weeks later they're running faster.

It sounds like snake oil, but it isn't. Just ask Bill for a peek into his bulging folder of thank-you letters and emails. A runner's success can never be guaranteed. Life happens to us all—we have to change jobs, we get injured, we're waylaid by a family health crisis . . . the list goes on and on. But the FIRST training program is more closely studied and more guaranteed than any other running program I have ever seen. What's more, you'll spend less time training than you are right now. You've got nothing to lose. It's a win-win program that has worked for hundreds of other runners, and there's no reason it can't work for you.

PREFACE

The first edition of *Run Less, Run Faster* elicited an overwhelming response: More than 7,500 messages from runners on six continents provided us with valuable feedback to the FIRST (Furman Institute of Running and Scientific Training) training programs. The daily messages from around the globe have given us insight into the challenges runners face whether they're training in the sweltering Philippines or South Florida, in subzero, snow-covered Canada or Scandinavia, in the desert sandstorms of Iraq, or on an oscillating ship in the Persian Gulf. Others have needed to deal with living in a town with no running track or traveling on business with access only to a hotel treadmill. Equally daunting are the problems that face a mother of five who must train between 4:00 and 5:30 a.m. or a second-shift worker who begins training at midnight. Many have special medical problems; others describe how professional obligations have left them sedentary for years and others want to know how to begin or enhance their training. Runners faced with all of these special challenges have sought advice from us on how to use the FIRST training program effectively.

We have responded to every message. In quite a few instances, an initial message has resulted in exchanges of questions and advice lasting several years. We have filed and kept notes on all of the inquiries. Those many questions, as well as our readers' reports of success and failure, provide the basis for this revised edition.

The popularity of the first edition gave us many opportunities to speak at race expos, clinics, and professional meetings. At those engagements we met many midpack runners, as well as noted authors and elite runners. These interactions enabled us to learn more about what runners seek and how we might better meet their needs.

In 2003, when the Running Institute was established, we declared that our mission was to promote lifelong participation in running and physical activity, while helping runners of all ages and abilities realize their potential through individually tailored training programs. Even though we had been providing such help to local runners for years, it was through the press that our message became global. Without a doubt, the article that Amby Burfoot wrote in the August 2005 edition of *Runner's World* ignited the interest of runners in the FIRST Training Programs. Runners still write that they began training with our program because of it. That article also appeared in multiple international editions of *Runner's World*; thus we began hearing immediately from runners in Australia, New Zealand, Southern Africa, the United Kingdom, Germany, and other European countries. The *Runner's World* article spawned a proliferation of articles in daily newspapers across the country including the *New York Times,* the *Chicago Tribune,* the *Wall Street Journal,* and magazines including *Bloomberg Businessweek, Men's Health, Women's Health, Parade,* and *National Geographic Adventurer,* all of which magnified interest in FIRST.

An intriguing opportunity growing out of this exposure is FIRST's collaboration with Running Buddy Sports in Bangalore, India. Running Buddy Sports is a venture established by Ashok Nath, Bhasker Sharma, and Rajesh Vetcha, all committed runners themselves, who came to Furman University in the summer of 2011 and were trained in all aspects of the FIRST program. Using FIRST training programs, these successful business executives plan to promote running in India and enable Indian runners to stay motivated, active, and injury free. Mass participation in competitive running is just beginning to grow in India, and FIRST is pleased to help encourage it.

We are excited about the opportunity to update our first edition because we are eager to share what we have learned. From the thousands of email messages, from the hundreds of runners who have traveled to Greenville, South Carolina, to visit us at Furman University, and from the hundreds of runners we have coached and the many conversations we've had with runners at race expos and clinics, we realized that there were important unanswered questions about the FIRST training programs in the first edition of *Run Less, Run Faster.* In this edition we address those questions. In addition, we have tweaked the tables and training programs based on runners' reports of their experience. Because of the international interest, we have also provided a metric version of all of our programs.

Don't be surprised if you find repeated mention of the key elements of the program: the importance of intensity, the integral role of cross training, the critical role that recovery plays, and the importance of pace selection and the avoidance of injuries. As anyone who has played on a high school or college team knows, that's what coaches do. Coaches want to make sure that athletes are getting the message and incorporating it in their training on a routine basis.

The core of the **FIRST 3plus2 Training Program** remains unchanged from the first edition—quality over quantity with individualized training goals for every run. While the first edition of the book focused on the research studies that convinced us of the program's efficacy, this second edition is focused on the practical aspects of using the workouts and reflects the thousands of success stories runners have shared with us. Nothing is more gratifying than receiving a heartwarming message from a runner describing how the FIRST training program enabled him or her to achieve a lifelong dream.

As I did in the first edition, I will represent my coauthors, Scott Murr and Ray Moss, as the voice of the book. As narrator, 1 will share with you our personal and professional experiences in exploring how to train efficiently.

Bill Pierce
October 2011

RUNNER'S WORLD.

RUN LESS
RUN FASTER

Training with Purpose

CHAPTER 1

THE FIRST 3PLUS2 TRAINING PROGRAM

In August 2005, Scott Infanger and Aaron Colangelo simultaneously read Amby Burfoot's article in *Runner's World* about the FIRST training program. As a result, they both became interested in the **3plus2** program. Amby chronicled the successes of the 25 participants in the 2004 FIRST marathon research study and profiled six runners who had achieved personal goals in the marathon with the program. Infanger and Colangelo both aspired to qualify for Boston by running a 3:10 marathon. Both submitted an application to be in our 2005 marathon training program study. Soon both were traveling from their respective homes in Nashville, Tennessee, and Washington, DC, to Furman University for their initial testing in the Molnar Human Performance Laboratory. They followed the FIRST 16-week marathon training program monitored by FIRST via email. After 15 weeks of faithfully following the program they traveled back to South Carolina for their posttraining program laboratory assessments. What would the data show? Had the targeted workouts resulted in an improvement? Would 3:10 be attainable? Because the faster times that they had seen in their training were consistent with their physiological test improvements, we told them that with smart pacing, a Boston qualification was possible, but it would require a focused effort. All of the participants in the study group participated in the Kiawah Island Marathon on the coast of South Carolina. Both Scott and Aaron ran smart races and qualified for Boston.

What we have learned over the past seven years and thousands of messages is that Scott's and Aaron's performances are not exceptional; rather, they are consistent with the successes of many using the FIRST training program. Most of the runners in our training studies improved both their race performances and their physiological profiles. Why do we think so many runners succeeded? Simply put, the workouts are designed with the purpose of improving speed and endurance. It all goes back to the concept of quality over quantity. Most runners measure their training by the number of miles run, rather than *how* those miles were run. Our **Training with Purpose** program provides structure and specific workouts tailored to the runner's current fitness level.

The basis of the program, described later in this chapter, is grounded on a sound philosophy and scientific principles. Is it for everyone? We don't think that any one training program is for everyone. Each individual responds differently to training programs (See "The Principles of Training" on page 12). History tells us that even elite runners have achieved their greatness using vastly different training methods. Is the FIRST training program the optimal way to train? We have never made that claim. We have said that it is a training program that works for many runners based on solid evidence. Not only from our studies that collected and examined physiological data, but more important, from those who have followed the training programs to racing successes.

Runners who've posted marathon times ranging from 2:40 to 6:00 hours tell us that the FIRST training program was central to their achievements. Many of the runners who say that they succeeded with the FIRST program had been injured in the past from programs that required running almost every day or focused on high mileage. The FIRST program provided them with a means to participate injury-free in the sport that had become painful drudgery for many. A large number reported to us that they have busy professional lives that don't permit them to run more often than the three key run workouts (an essential part of the FIRST training program) and, furthermore, that they were able to achieve their goals—typically, a Boston qualification—with the FIRST marathon training program. Numerous clubs around the country have written us to say that their clubs use this program because the specific structure of the workouts makes it easy to provide each club member with an individualized goal for each workout. We have learned that runners are disciplined and dedicated and like structure and accountability. The FIRST training program gives you a specific distance and pace for each workout based on your current level of running fitness.

The FIRST training program is designed to produce optimal results with limited running. We have compressed our collective knowledge, experience, and research into a method that provides specific workouts laid out in 12- and 16-week training schedules for races from 5Ks to marathons (see Tables 5.1–5.5 in Chapter 5). These efficient and effective schedules have been tested with runners of wide-ranging abilities. Along with the training schedules, we include answers to many of the most frequently asked questions that we have received from runners around the world.

This book is designed with a philosophy similar to that of the FIRST training program. The chapters provide the essentials for becoming fitter and faster. We realize that it is unlikely that anyone has time to devote to an extensive regimen of strength training, flexibility, and cross-training. Likewise, we know that lengthy chapters on the complex topics of nutrition, environmental factors, and injuries can be more daunting to the reader than helpful. We have attempted to give you a practical number of important exercises that will keep you strong, flexible, and fit while not requiring much time. These basic exercises will enhance your running and contribute to keeping you healthy and injury free. By paring the information about nutrition to simple guidelines, we believe that you can become a healthy eater and a well-fueled runner by following our advice. Similarly, the information about how to cope with the heat and cold can aid your training. Most important, we wish to help you stay healthy. All of our workouts and exercises are designed to help you avoid injury while recognizing that running is a physical activity that requires repetitive movements of impact that contribute to overuse.

WHAT IS THE FIRST PHILOSOPHY?

At the heart of the FIRST philosophy is the belief that most runners do not train with purpose. When we ask runners to share their typical training week and the objective of each run, they can't explain why they do what they do. When they don't have a training plan that incorporates different distances, paces, and recoveries, they don't reach their potential. Nor do they garner maximum benefits from their investment in training time. The FIRST program makes running easier and more accessible, limits overtraining and burnout, and substantially cuts the risk of injury while producing faster race times. By focusing on efficient, purposeful training, the FIRST program enables runners to meet their goal of running faster without sacrificing job, health, family, and friends.

THE FIRST 3PLUS2 TRAINING PROGRAM AND ITS COMPONENTS

Three quality runs each week plus two cross-training workouts are the foundation of the breakthrough FIRST approach. The three runs—the track repeats, the tempo run, and the long run—are designed to work together to improve endurance, lactate-threshold running pace, and leg speed. For each run, the FIRST program prescribes specific paces and distances that are based on a runner's current level of running fitness. The three quality runs including prescribed paces and distances are described in detail in Chapter 5.

Having a specific goal for each training run is another of the program's innovations—when we ask most runners what they're hoping to accomplish on a given run, they answer with a blank stare. If you don't know what you're training toward, how can you possibly get there?

The FIRST program's prescribed paces are usually reported by runners as being faster than their normal running speed. Generally, this is because our **Training with Purpose** philosophy favors quality over quantity, intensity over frequency, fast running over the accumulation of miles. If you want to run faster, you need to train faster. In addition to running less, what sets the FIRST program apart from other training programs is that it emphasizes a faster pace for the long runs. In our studies, we've discovered that focusing on a designated, demanding pace for the long runs prepares runners physiologically and mentally for racing, particularly for the marathon. Studies in various sports show that competitive practices produce more focused competitors in games and competitions. The focus necessary to complete each FIRST key run workout makes runners mentally stronger in races.

The physiological value of this faster running is that it increases the muscles' ability to metabolize lactate. Why is this important? The process associated with the accumulation of excess lactate inhibits aerobic energy availability for muscular action. By training at a higher intensity, the muscle adapts to the increased energy demand by developing the ability to use lactate as an energy source, rather than have it accumulate in the muscles and blood.

The FIRST Training Program differs from the typical running program not only by its emphasis on intensity but also by building in more recovery time between running workouts. Without sufficient recovery, you'll find it difficult to have quality workouts. Muscles need time to recover from the stress of hard workouts. Stressing specific muscle fibers repeatedly, day after day, in the same pattern causes accumulated fatigue. In other words, running 6 miles 5 days a week results in muscular fatigue, not muscular adaptation. However, using those same muscle fibers for a different type of activity will permit recovery and recharging of the muscle's energy stores (glycogen). You can engage in another aerobic activity and reap the cardiorespiratory benefits while the muscle fibers used in running are recharging for the next hard running workout. Chapter 7 explains further the importance of rest and recovery.

Most other running programs ignore the benefits of cross-training in favor of running more miles. FIRST's cross-training workouts not only enhance fitness but also add variety, which ultimately reduces vulnerability to overuse injuries. Plus, your training will be more interesting. Cross-training workouts at prescribed intensities increase blood flow around muscles, which in turn increases the muscles' ability to utilize oxygen and fat as energy sources for exercise. Using fat as an energy source spares the limited stores of carbohydrates (glycogen). Therefore, cross-training provides the same benefit as the additional running miles of other typical running programs. In Chapter 6, the **3plus2** training program's cross-training workouts are described in detail.

WHERE'S THE PROOF?

In 2003, when we established the Running Institute, we were convinced from our own experiences that these three running workouts, coupled with vigorous cross-training, would help runners improve both their race times and overall fitness. We were eager to conduct training studies with a variety of runners to evaluate our **Training with Purpose** running philosophy by testing our **3plus2** program. We had designed the programs to help runners train effectively and efficiently and to avoid overtraining and injury. But could we prove that they were, in fact, doing all these things?

Exercise science studies testing the effectiveness of training regimens typically are conducted in laboratories where potentially confounding variables can be controlled. We stewed over how to design our studies. Our goal was to find a program that would enable us to generalize the results to the typical runner, not just male college freshmen. Many research studies use male college freshmen as subjects because professors have easy access to them. We wanted to test our programs on "real" runners—fast, slow, male, female, young, old, novices, or race veterans—performing their training without direct supervision. That required our giving up control. We also wanted to find out if our program worked for real runners in spite of the program's restrictions: finding an accessible running track, having a measured running course for tempo and long runs, and being able to maintain a specific pace for a workout.

For 3 consecutive years we conducted studies each with 25 participants, men and women from all over the country ranging in ages from 23 to 63, who agreed to follow the FIRST training program for 16 weeks. Each study began with the participants being tested in the laboratory to assess their fitness. After following the 16-week training program, they returned for repeat testing. In addition to the laboratory assessments, in the latter two studies, the participants also ran a marathon. In all three studies, the runners showed significant improvement over the 16 weeks of training. All three variables—maximal oxygen consumption, running speed at lactate threshold, and running speed at peak oxygen consumption critical to running performance had been enhanced by following a three-quality-runs-per-week training program. We now had data to support our personal experiences. And most important to the runners themselves, each improved on at least one of the running performance variables. A summary of the studies' results is reported later in this chapter.

The three-quality-runs-per-week training program enabled all of the first-time marathoners to finish, very much satisfied with their performance times. More impressive were the personal best times recorded by more than 70 percent of the veteran marathoners. Running only 3 days a week, coupled with two cross-training workouts, enabled even veteran marathoners who were accustomed to running 5 or 6 days a week to improve their physiological profiles from the laboratory assessment, as well as to improve their marathon performances.

The studies supplied strong proof that the training programs were effective and led us to write *Run Less, Run Faster*. Yet we believe that the evidence provided by the many successes reported over the past 5 years is even stronger proof that the FIRST training approach is effective. Having runners follow the program on their own, rather than have us monitor their workouts and provide them feedback, is a strong endorsement that the program can be used without direct coaching. The reports from those who used our program and achieved a personal best or a Boston qualifying time indicate that runners across a wide range of abilities, ages, experience, both female and male, from six continents got fitter and faster.

Training with Purpose means having workouts designed to specifically target the determinants of running performance. These studies and the countless success stories indicate that our **3plus2** training program is not an empty promise. Runners tend to have more confidence in methods that other runners have used successfully. The FIRST training program also provides the structure and accountability that runners like by specifying both distance and pace for each workout, so there is a clear measure of performance for each training run. Running 6 miles is one thing, running 6 miles only 30 seconds slower than 10K pace is quite another.

Can All Runners Benefit from the FIRST Training Program?

Our research studies say *yes* for age-group runners; however, we have not tested it with national and world-class runners. This training program was designed for regular runners aspiring to improve their running. The FIRST training program has been used to improve performances by 5-hour marathoners and sub-3-hour marathoners, by those preparing for their first 5K or marathon, and by beginners in their early 20s as well as veterans in their 70s and 80s. In addition, the **3plus2** training program is extremely flexible and can be adjusted to fit the needs of all types of runners, from those who have limited time to train to those who make training a major focus in their lives.

Results of the Three Studies

Pre- and post-training, three variables were compared to determine the effects of the 16-week training program: (1) VO_2max, (2) running speed at lactate threshold, and (3) running speed at peak VO_2. The results are displayed in the summary table (Table 1.1). You can see that as a group in all three studies, the runners showed improvement over the 16 weeks of training on all three variables related to running performance, all statistically significant. Individually, every runner improved on at least one of the running performance variables.

Table 1.1

Summary of Results from Three FIRST Studies

(Runners in the 2003 study did not run a marathon at the end of the study. They were assessed only in our lab.)

	2003	2004	2005
Females	7	10	8
Males	15	12	9
Ages	23–63 years	25–56 years	24–52 years
Average Age	F = 41.7 M = 40.1	F = 34.8 M = 36.7	F = 35 M = 35.4
% Improvement of VO_2 max	4.8	4.2	5.4
% Improvement of Running Speed at Lactate Threshold	4.4	2.3	5.6
% Improvement of Running Speed at Peak VO_2	7.9	2.4	2.1
Range of Marathon Finish Times for Females		3:56–4:44	3:41–4:49
Average Marathon Finish Times for Females		Median = 4:17:02 Mean = 4:20:42	Median = 3:56:18 Mean = 4:02:22
Range of Marathon Finish Times for Males		2:56–4:51	2:57–4:19
Average Marathon Finish Times for Males		Median = 3:46:19 Mean = 3:49:23	Median = 3:42:51 Mean = 3:35:24
Number of First-Time Marathon Finishers		8 (3F, 5M)	3 (2M, 1F)
Average Time of First-Time Marathoners		F (3) = 4:03:07 M (5) = 3:48:49	F (1) = 4:03:34 M (2) = 3:46:22
Number of Personal Best Times (for those who had run a marathon previously)		7 of 13 (53.8%)	12 of 14 (85.7%)

THE PRINCIPLES OF TRAINING

There are five primary principles of training that apply to runners. These five principles should be incorporated into any training program. FIRST training programs adhere to these five basic training principles:

Principle #1

Progressive Overload: The gradual increase of training stress will cause the body to adapt in response to that overload. These adaptations occur at the cellular level, and this adaptation process will continue as long as the overload doesn't overwhelm the system. That is why the additional stress— increased exercise time and intensity—must increase gradually.

Principle #2

Specificity: The improvement from training will be specific to the type of training. Specificity applies to the mode (type) of exercise, intensity (speed or pace), and duration (distance or total time run). Obviously, to become a good runner you need to run. The question is how much of your training needs to be mode-specific. The FIRST program requires a smaller percentage of your total training to be running than other running programs. As we explain throughout the book, our experience and research show that a high level of fitness and running success can be achieved with running three times a week.

The FIRST training approach adheres to the principle of specificity for intensity. We advocate that to run faster, you must incorporate faster running into your training. Runners report that the FIRST training paces are challenging. Runners also report that training hard helps them race faster than running more frequently in training. Pace-specific training is the primary basis of FIRST training.

Principle #3

Individual Differences: Runners will soon find that they may improve more than their training partners and that others improve faster than they do. Individuals are different in their anatomies and physiologies.

REAL RUNNER REPORT

Dear Bill Pierce,

I would like to thank you for the amazing training program that you have developed.

Last June I ran my first marathon in South Bend, Indiana, and I was able to achieve my goal of finishing under 4 hours. I finished at 3:55:03.

The problem was that by the end of my training I was feeling tired, and 2 weeks before the race, both of my knees were killing me. My orthopedic specialist told me to forget about the marathon and take some time off from running. I was devastated. I was running an average of 40–46 miles a week. I guess at the age of 36, my body couldn't handle all those miles well. I knew that I had to follow a different program for my second marathon.

My goal was to qualify for Boston. That meant that I had to shave 10 minutes off my time. I came across your program, and after reading the book, I decided that it made complete sense. I followed it religiously. Never skipped a run or cross-training workout. I did all the stretch and strength exercises that you have in the book. I was on a mission. The week before my marathon, I felt ready, but also the weird thing was that nothing was hurting me. I felt as light as a feather.

On January 17th, 2010, I ran the P.F. Chang's Rock and Roll Marathon in Arizona. I'm proud to announce that my time was 3:43:09. I qualified for Boston, but my biggest accomplishment was that I ran almost identical splits. My first half was 9 seconds faster than the second half of the race. I felt strong throughout the whole marathon. It has been almost a week and I feel fully recovered. Nothing is hurting, nothing is sore, and I can't wait to start running again.

I tell everybody about your book, and a lot of my friends have been inspired by my success. I couldn't have done it without you.

Thank you from the bottom of my heart.

Christina Kostouros
Personal Trainer
Crown Point, Indiana

FOLLOW-UP MESSAGE:

Your book is like the Bible in my house.

I just completed the Boston Marathon. I felt strong throughout the whole race. My time was 3:38:37, and I was extremely happy to qualify for Boston in Boston.

Thanks again.

Individuals respond differently to the same training regimen. It is important that you realize that the most important factor that you consider is your own progress—where you are now, as opposed to where you were or where you will be 3 months from now. There will always be others who are fitter and faster and others who are less fit and slower. The principle of individual differences also applies to rest and recovery.

Principle #4

Law of Diminishing Returns: One of the benefits of being a novice is that your early progress is substantial. As you progress through the training programs and you get fitter and faster, you are approaching your optimal performance. As you near that point, small improvements come from lots of hard training, as opposed to the large improvements that came from moderate training when you were first beginning.

Principle #5

Reversibility: Use it or lose it! The gains that you make can be lost if you stop training. Consistency is the key to fitness.

The FIRST program encourages regular year-round training. That is one of the attractive features of running three times per week. Runners do not feel overwhelmed and overstressed with the rigors of daily running, which causes some to stop running for long periods. Interruptions in regular physical activity cause a loss of fitness that leads us to try to make up for those losses too fast once we return to training. The training does not have to be at full intensity year-round; low to moderate intensity can help you maintain fitness and not be susceptible to the stress and injuries that come from sudden increases in physical activity.

CHAPTER 2

REALISTIC GOALS

Runners who attend FIRST Retreats and those who write to us want to know if their goals are realistic. They want us to tell them what race times they are capable of running now and what race times they can expect to run in the future. Based on their training times and, in the case of those who have visited our laboratory, their physiological profile, we can give a fairly accurate estimate of their race finish times. However, we don't have a crystal ball and cannot provide a future prediction with certainty. That's why you enter races.

There are many variables that determine race performances; not all of them are nicely quantified on a computer printout from a metabolic system. However, the more data from both lab and field tests we have to consider, the better we can help the runner set realistic goals.

In particular, marathon time prediction is difficult. Time prediction for shorter races, from 5Ks to half-marathons, is fairly predictable, assuming that the runner chooses a realistic pace and has prepared appropriately for the distance. Perhaps the allure of the marathon is related to its uncertainty. We love games that go down to the final minute of play with the outcome undetermined. Uncertainty is the element of sport that contributes to its popularity. I believe that the same is true of the marathon. I am seldom, if ever, surprised by the outcome of a 5K, 8K, 10K, 10 mile, or half-marathon race. I know within seconds what I will be able to run. With the marathon, it's a mystery. Even during the race, whether you are halfway, at 20 or 24 miles, you won't know what is going to happen next.

There are many variables that affect marathon performance. You battle physical challenges such as maintaining core temperature and fuel stores, muscular fatigue, and orthopedic stress all the way to the finish line. Any one of those factors can undermine great preparation and a good performance over many miles. Changes in environmental conditions, such as temperature, headwinds or humidity, also may spoil your best laid plans.

Marathoners who fail to achieve their goal finish times immediately begin to question their preparation and training. In many cases, their preparation was good and appropriate, but they may have been unlucky because one of the many variables noted above was not right on that day. However, setting an unrealistic finish-time goal that is just a couple of minutes too fast, particularly in the marathon, will lead to a too fast early pace that will undermine good preparation and a great effort.

Why is it that runners are disappointed with race finish times? Often it is not because of a poor performance, but it's the result of their having set unrealistic goals. For example, a runner who just finished a 10K in 40:30 might be despondent because she had hoped to run under 40:00. It may be that she just ran a superb race. That is, based on her 5K and half-marathon times, her predicted 10K time was 41:00, which means she ran 5 seconds per mile faster than what was predicted. She just had a remarkable performance from what had to be a great effort, but her expectations prevented her from enjoying and appreciating it.

The question is: Why and how did she establish 40:00 as her target finish time for the 10K? Most likely her disappointment is a result of wanting to be a "30 something" 10K runner, just as runners want to be a "3 something" or "2 something" marathoner. If I had been coaching her, I would have told her that based on her recent performances at these other race distances and on her training paces, that running 10 seconds per mile faster than what was predicted was unlikely and trying to do so would likely result in her fading over the last couple of miles. I would have said let's set three goals for your 10K: (1) 41:15, an acceptable run representing a good effort; (2) under 41:00, a very good performance and faster than predicted; and (3) under 40:45, an outstanding effort and performance.

As it was, she had an outstanding effort and performance, but was disappointed because she did not have a realistic goal. She could have benefited from good coaching advice. That's why we have placed this important topic so early in this book.

Of course, we want to encourage runners to challenge themselves and identify ambitious goals. However, running too fast early in the race because you chose an overly ambitious, unrealistic goal almost always leads to dire consequences in the second half of the race. You'll be disheartened when an outstanding performance is unsatisfying because you chose an arbitrary and unrealistic goal.

I find that many of the runners applying to FIRST for coaching have unrealistic goals. At least, they are unrealistic in the short term. They may be able to reach their goals with steady and wise training over a period of two years. Many expect miracles in 16 weeks. These unrealistic goal times result when runners select them arbitrarily, usually round numbers, or in many cases, a qualifying time such as that for the Boston Marathon. The way in which FIRST helps runners set realistic goals is just as valuable as our individually tailored training programs.

How do runners undermine their own performance? Consider this example. A runner with a 5K race finish time of 22:00 has a predicted marathon time of 3:34:05 (using Table 2.1, starting on page 26). If the runner sets 3:30 as a goal, he or she will need to run nearly 10 seconds faster per mile than the pace required to run a 3:34:05. Attempting to run 10 seconds per mile faster for 26.2 miles than what your current fitness level indicates will most likely result in a disappointing finish with your questioning what element was missing in your training program. The only thing missing was a realistic goal.

REALISTIC GOALS: THE ESSENTIALS

How to Select Your Goal Finish Time

• Use the time from your most recent race (5K, 10K, half-marathon or marathon) to determine a reasonable estimate or target time for one of the other distances (use Table 2.1).

• For marathoners, go to the Boston tables in Chapter 15 and review the criteria that indicate if each qualifying time is realistic for you. Those training times are good predictors of race performance.

• Know when it is wise to redefine your goals in either direction. Be objective about your training progress and apply all of the above criteria, including your ability to attain the target training paces for your key run workouts and races to determine if your goal is realistic.

REALISTIC GOALS: Q AND A

Q. How does the selection of the goal finish time affect your performance?

A. Selecting a goal finish time that's too ambitious will cause you to run too fast at the start. That fast start will likely result in a slower pace in the latter part of the race and a disappointing finish time.

Q. If my 10K time predicts a 3:13 marathon, is it okay to set 3:10 as my goal?

A. Running 3 minutes faster than your predicted marathon finish time means running 7 seconds faster per mile than the pace that is presumably representative of your current fitness level. For most marathoners, running 7 seconds per mile faster for the entire distance would be challenging and most likely not realistic. Trying to do so could lead to a disappointing finish time.

Q. Would it be reasonable to expect an improvement over a 16- to 18-week training period that would make the 3:10 in the previous question possible?

A. Absolutely, that's why we train. While there are no guarantees, due to numerous variables (weather, course, personal health, etc.), a good marathon training program can produce that result. We have had runners in our training programs make much bigger improvements. For the purpose of setting a revised goal, don't assume that improvement has occurred without confirmation from a shorter race or improved training times. In particular, we rely on long run training times to judge a runner's improvement and his or her potential marathon performance; we use tempo training times to determine a runner's improvement and his or her potential 5K and 10K goal times. Your improvement will depend on the type of training that you have done in the past.

Q. What distance is the best predictor? What if the 5K and 10K predict different marathon finish times?

A. The distance closest to the planned race distance is going to be the better predictor, assuming that the races were run under similar conditions. That is, a 10K is a better predictor of your marathon finish time than a 5K race finish time and a half-marathon finish time will be a better marathon predictor than the 10K time.

If your 5K predicts a faster marathon time than what you are able to run, it is an indication that you have more speed than endurance and you need to concentrate on your longer runs. Conversely, if your marathon finish time predicts a faster 5K time than you are able to run, then you need to work on speed and leg turnover.

Q. Are the prediction tables accurate for everyone?

A. Individuals differ in their abilities. Some runners have more speed than endurance and vice versa. For some runners their 5K finish times will predict a faster marathon than what they can run, while for others, their marathon times are faster than what their 5K times predict.

Q. Are there differences in the tables for men and women?

A. Generally, women will run faster for longer distances and men faster for shorter distances. That is, if you have a male and a female with the same 5K time, the female will likely run a faster marathon than the male. Conversely, if you have a male and a female with the same marathon time, the male will likely run a faster 5K than the female. From reviewing race results and single-age world records, we have found that older women (55 and older) tend to slow at an accelerated rate as compared to that for men. Is this inherent for females or is it a matter of culture? Will these race results and records change as more women with a longer history of competing become older?

Q. Does age make a difference in the prediction tables?

A. Aging runners usually have more endurance than speed. If a 55-year-old runner and 20-year-old runner have the same 5K time, it is likely that the 55-year-old would run the faster half- or full marathon. Conversely, if the 55-year-old and the 20-year-old had the same marathon time, the 20-year-old would likely have a faster 5K time. Older runners tend to be more economical and younger runners have more speed.

Q. How does the course profile affect the goal finish time?

A. The fastest road racing times in the world at all distances have been set on flat courses with few turns (Berlin, Rotterdam, Chicago). Hills, turns, rough or uneven surfaces all tend to slow the pace. While many runners will say that a flat course is boring and that they welcome a change to the repetitive, concentrated muscular contractions, there is a time cost for those changes. There are no clear measures to determine the time cost of specific elevation changes. Rolling hills may make the course more interesting and fun to run; they will not contribute to a faster finish time. Often, there are Web site forums where veteran runners of a race will estimate what the time difference is for a specific race course as compared to that for a flat course. Those postings by past participants in the race usually provide more helpful and accurate descriptions of a race course and its difficulty than the race's Web site.

Q. Does my predicted finish time from the tables assume that there will be some elevation changes in the race?

A. Assume that the finish time prediction is valid if the race that you are using to predict your finish time at another distance is similar in terrain to that race. That is, if you ran a hilly 5K and you are using that race time to predict your half-marathon time on a hilly course, it is likely to be a reasonable predictor. However, if you ran a perfectly flat 10K and are using that time to predict your finish time on a hilly marathon course, then you should add time to that prediction to compensate for the additional time required for running the hills, depending on the length and steepness.

Q. How do environmental conditions influence goal finish time?

A. Ideal racing temperatures for most runners range from 40 to 60 degrees Fahrenheit (5 to 16 degrees Celsius). A general estimate is that for every degree above 60 degrees F you will slow by 1 second per mile in the marathon. Of course, there are wide individual variations based on sweat rates and body size. Smaller runners, who are able to dissipate heat better than larger runners, have the advantage in the heat, but are disadvantaged in colder temperatures. The extra energy cost of maintaining body temperature depends on the length of the race and one's body size. Even light winds on a cool day (less than 60 degrees F or 15 degrees C) can increase demands on the body for maintaining normal body temperature. Needless to say, having a race day with the ideal temperature, humidity, and winds is a rare treat for the runner. Look what those once-in-a-century ideal conditions produced at the 2011 Boston Marathon. Unpredictable environmental conditions are just one additional factor that makes determining realistic goals a challenge. Do not fool yourself by thinking that you will defy environmental conditions and their effects on physiology; you won't.

Q. As I get older my race times are slower. Is there a way to determine comparable times at my present age to those that I ran when I was younger?

A. Yes, World Masters Athletics (WMA) has developed tables that adjust performances for aging. The age-graded factors and standards were developed based on the world records for that single year age. Look at the results from the St. George Marathon and you will see not only runners' finish clock times and chip times, but also their age-graded percentage. This percentage represents a comparison of an individual's performance to the world record performance by a runner of that age. By using this method, runners can compare their performances, or percentages, to other runners or to their own performances at a younger age. It is a method for aging runners to set realistic goals.

For example, a 50-year-old female with a marathon time of 3:55 can go to Appendix C (Road Age Factors WMA 2010) and convert that 3:55 to an equivalent time for a marathon run at prime marathon age (21–29) for females by multiplying her 3:55 (235 minutes) by the 0.8420 factor for 50-year-old female marathoners. That produces a 3:17:52 age-adjusted performance time.

Some races have begun to provide age-graded performance standards. What this means is that finish times are adjusted for the assumed performance decrement (percentage of increase in race time) based on age. Some races even present awards based on age-adjusted performance times. Younger runners no doubt see this method of adjusting times as noncompetitive, while older runners see it as eminently fair!

Q. How do I determine my age-graded performance level percentage?

A. Use the Road Age Standards WMA 2010 in Appendix B to find your age-graded standard and then divide the standard by your race time. For example, a 60-year-old male with a 5K time of 20:00 would divide the standard of 16:02 for a 60-year-old male by 20:00. The result (962 seconds/1200 seconds) would be 80.2 percent. That percentage could be compared to the age-graded percentages of performances run at earlier ages or with other runners of different ages.

Q. How do I convert my current race time to an equivalent race time at an earlier age?

A. Use Road Age Factors WMA 2010 in Appendix C for males to find your age factor. Multiply that age factor by your current race time to determine your equivalent race time at your prime-age time. For example, that 60-year-old male whose time is 20:00 for the 5K would multiply that 20:00 by the age factor of .8043 and see that his 20:00 5K at age 60 is equivalent to a 16:05 at prime 5K performance age for males, which is the 22- to 28-year old age group.

Q. What is the prime performance age?

A. You can see in Road Age Factors WMA 2010 in Appendix C that the prime age for running performances varies for males and females, as well as varying for the different distances. The age-adjusted times are based on world records for a single age. Males tend to run world-class times at an older age than females. Male runners also perform at their prime at an older age for longer distances. There are no adjustments in finish times for male marathoners until age 36, but 5K and 10K runners have finish times adjusted for age beginning at 29 and half-marathoners at age 32. Females begin receiving age adjustments for all distances beginning at around age 30.

REALISTIC GOALS: THE SCIENCE

In the seminal book *The Lore of Running,* Tim Noakes, MD, claims that the best predictor of running performance at any distance is a running time test, rather than a laboratory assessment of physiological measures. Marathoners can utilize various prediction formulas based on their race times at shorter distances. Numerous prediction tables for distances from 800 meters to ultramarathons exist. All of these tables assume appropriate race-specific training on the part of the runner. The table at the end of this chapter (Table 2.1) provides comparable race times for four popular race distances. These equivalent performances were developed by calculating race finish times as percentages of the world records.

An Early Fast Pace Has Consequences

Running authors Bob Glover and Pete Schuder cautioned that if marathon runners are more than 2 minutes faster than their target half-marathon split, then they have blown their marathon and will suffer for it over the last few miles. Marathoners commonly refer to a dramatic slowing of pace in the marathon as "hitting the wall." Speculations about the causes of hitting the wall include a variety of physiological explanations. Through marathon preparation and proper nutrition, you can increase your muscle's glycogen stores to high levels. My coauthor Ray Moss reminds runners that the amount of glycogen you have stored is all that the muscles have available to use throughout the race. Improper pacing will deplete glycogen stores and you'll hit the wall before you finish the marathon. David Costill, noted exercise physiologist and running researcher, stated that hitting the wall is simply a matter of poor pacing. It should be noted that Stephen Seiler, an exercise scientist at the Institute for Sport at Agder College in Norway, explains that "An early misuse of pace results in a lactic acid accumulation that cannot be eliminated without a subsequent decrease in speed." Furthermore, he reported that for each second gained by going under optimal pace in the first half of a race, 2 seconds are lost in the second half due to premature fatigue.

No matter how strongly we advocate not running the first half of the race too fast, most runners fail to follow that advice. There are good reasons for their failure: (1) the excitement of race day causes the adrenaline to flow and that exuberance causes the runner to lose the ability to judge pacing, (2) having runners surround you at the start of the race also distorts pacing, that is, you are just running with the crowd so it doesn't feel too fast, (3) when you are rested from your prerace taper, your target pace feels easier in the early part of the race than in training, and (4) for reasons 1, 2, and 3 you get the sense that *this is my day* and you begin mentally revising your goal finish time downward. However, during the second half you begin to feel fatigued because you have withdrawn your stored energy in the muscle cells too rapidly and you begin mile after mile revising your goal finish time upward. Your marathoning experience will be much more satisfying and pleasant if you have a strong finish than if you fade over the last few miles, even if you were to achieve the same finish time in the two different scenarios.

We have analyzed tens of thousands of race finish times and found that only about 2 percent of runners run the second half of the race in the same time as the first half. Run the first half too fast and you slow down at a much faster rate in the second half. Run the first half too slowly and you can't make up the time in the second half. We strongly believe that running even splits is a desirable goal and a realistic one for 5Ks, 10Ks, and half-marathons. It is far more difficult to maintain a constant pace over 26.2 miles. For the marathon, you should strive to keep the time disparity between the two halves less than 2 minutes, but a disparity of 5 minutes is common and can still produce a successful marathon. For example, 1:32 for the first half and around 1:35–1:37 for the second half. When the disparity between the two halves becomes greater than 5 minutes, the marathoner has failed to achieve the near-optimal finish time and reach her or his potential.

AGING AND FIRST TRAINING

While the FIRST training programs were designed and have been effective for runners of all ages, they have been particularly popular with older runners. As runners age they need more recovery and that typically leads to reduced training volume. Much research is being conducted on older runners. Whether the research is focused on mental or physical functioning, the results are clear that the key to good health and performance is to stay active and to do so consistently, so as to stave off the deterioration that we once thought inevitable. Let me be clear that running performance will decline with aging, save for those who begin running late in life. However, the performance reductions predicted in the literature are being defied by a generation of runners who have maintained their intense training for decades.

Aging runners rarely escape without injury. As connective tissue becomes less supple and more susceptible to injury, tendinitis from inflammation is a common occurrence. After an injury that might sideline the older runner for weeks or months, fitness is lost and the attempt to regain it too fast leads to another injury and a vicious cycle of injury and recovery develops. This can lead to a more serious injury or a loss of motivation, both of which can lead to one's becoming a former runner. That status contributes to weight gain and accompanying medical conditions associated with being sedentary. It's important to find a way through treatment and rehabilitation of an injury to maintain your fitness.

As runners' times begin to slow, there may be a loss of motivation to train intensely. Dr. Hirofumi Tanaka, an exercise physiologist at the University of Texas, in a *New York Times* article about aging recommended training intensely to improve oxygen consumption. In the same *Times* article by Gina Kolata, Dr. Steven Hawkins, an exercise physiologist at the University of Southern California, said that when you have to choose between hard and often, choose hard. He added that "high performance is really determined more by intensity than volume. Sometimes when you're older, something has to give. You can't have both so you have to cut back on the volume. You need more rest days." These two exercise physiologists' advice echo the philosophy central to the FIRST training program.

Training consistently is the key for aging runners because it is much easier to maintain fitness than to get fit as you age. While the times on the watch may represent slower performances, it is the intensity of the effort that matters. Yes, performances will decline, but serious training will reduce these inevitable decrements by 50 percent or more. Runners who continue to train seriously will typically experience racing decrements less than 1 percent per year from their late thirties to mid-forties. The slower performance times will most likely occur sooner in the shorter races—5K to 10K—than in the longer races. Marathoners can still run their best times in their late 30s and early 40s. For runners who sustain their training, performance losses in the 0.5 percent to 1 percent range can be expected from the mid-forties to mid-fifties. The slowing of performance times accelerates after age 55 with annual performance decrements ranging from 1 percent to 2.5 percent.

Bob Dylan had it right—"the times they are a-changin'." We suspect that the aging literature about runners will be completely rewritten as the baby boomers march into old age. FIRST is proud that its programs have enabled runners in their sixties, seventies, and eighties, whose old ways of training had led to slower times and a loss of motivation, to report a renewed excitement with their training along with improved age-group times. The masters age-adjusted tables in Appendices B and C provide age-adjusted times so that older runners can determine their running times' equivalences to those run at a younger age. These tables can be valuable in helping to set realistic goals.

Table 2.1

Race Prediction Table (Equivalent Performances)

Use the table to determine comparable performance times for four popular racing distances. The comparability assumes that you are properly trained for that distance.

5K	10K	HALF-MARATHON	MARATHON
0:16:00	0:33:29	1:14:10	2:35:42
0:16:10	0:33:49	1:14:56	2:37:19
0:16:20	0:34:10	1:15:42	2:38:57
0:16:30	0:34:31	1:16:29	2:40:34
0:16:40	0:34:52	1:17:15	2:42:11
0:16:50	0:35:13	1:18:01	2:43:48
0:17:00	0:35:34	1:18:48	2:45:26
0:17:10	0:35:55	1:19:34	2:47:03
0:17:20	0:36:16	1:20:20	2:48:40
0:17:30	0:36:37	1:21:07	2:50:18
0:17:40	0:36:58	1:21:53	2:51:55
0:17:50	0:37:19	1:22:40	2:53:32
0:18:00	0:37:40	1:23:26	2:55:10
0:18:10	0:38:01	1:24:12	2:56:47
0:18:20	0:38:21	1:24:59	2:58:24
0:18:30	0:38:42	1:25:45	3:00:02
0:18:40	0:39:03	1:26:31	3:01:39
0:18:50	0:39:24	1:27:18	3:03:16
0:19:00	0:39:45	1:28:04	3:04:54
0:19:10	0:40:06	1:28:50	3:06:31
0:19:20	0:40:27	1:29:37	3:08:08
0:19:30	0:40:48	1:30:23	3:09:45
0:19:40	0:41:09	1:31:09	3:11:23
0:19:50	0:41:30	1:31:56	3:13:00
0:20:00	0:41:51	1:32:42	3:14:37
0:20:10	0:42:12	1:33:28	3:16:15
0:20:20	0:42:32	1:34:15	3:17:52
0:20:30	0:42:53	1:35:01	3:19:29
0:20:40	0:43:14	1:35:47	3:21:07
0:20:50	0:43:35	1:36:34	3:22:44
0:21:00	0:43:56	1:37:20	3:24:21
0:21:10	0:44:17	1:38:07	3:25:59

5K	10K	HALF-MARATHON	MARATHON
0:21:20	0:44:38	1:38:53	3:27:36
0:21:30	0:44:59	1:39:39	3:29:13
0:21:40	0:45:20	1:40:26	3:30:51
0:21:50	0:45:41	1:41:12	3:32:28
0:22:00	0:46:02	1:41:58	3:34:05
0:22:10	0:46:23	1:42:45	3:35:42
0:22:20	0:46:44	1:43:31	3:37:20
0:22:30	0:47:04	1:44:17	3:38:57
0:22:40	0:47:25	1:45:04	3:40:34
0:22:50	0:47:46	1:45:50	3:42:12
0:23:00	0:48:07	1:46:36	3:43:49
0:23:10	0:48:28	1:47:23	3:45:26
0:23:20	0:48:49	1:48:09	3:47:04
0:23:30	0:49:10	1:48:55	3:48:41
0:23:40	0:49:31	1:49:42	3:50:18
0:23:50	0:49:52	1:50:28	3:51:56
0:24:00	0:50:13	1:51:14	3:53:33
0:24:10	0:50:34	1:52:01	3:55:10
0:24:20	0:50:55	1:52:47	3:56:48
0:24:30	0:51:16	1:53:34	3:58:25
0:24:40	0:51:36	1:54:20	4:00:02
0:24:50	0:51:57	1:55:06	4:01:39
0:25:00	0:52:18	1:55:53	4:03:17
0:25:10	0:52:39	1:56:39	4:04:54
0:25:20	0:53:00	1:57:25	4:06:31
0:25:30	0:53:21	1:58:12	4:08:09
0:25:40	0:53:42	1:58:58	4:09:46
0:25:50	0:54:03	1:59:44	4:11:23
0:26:00	0:54:24	2:00:31	4:13:01
0:26:10	0:54:45	2:01:17	4:14:38
0:26:20	0:55:06	2:02:03	4:16:15
0:26:30	0:55:27	2:02:50	4:17:53

5K	10K	HALF-MARATHON	MARATHON
0:26:40	0:55:48	2:03:36	4:19:30
0:26:50	0:56:08	2:04:22	4:21:07
0:27:00	0:56:29	2:05:09	4:22:44
0:27:10	0:56:50	2:05:55	4:24:22
0:27:20	0:57:11	2:06:42	4:25:59
0:27:30	0:57:32	2:07:28	4:27:36
0:27:40	0:57:53	2:08:14	4:29:14
0:27:50	0:58:14	2:09:01	4:30:51
0:28:00	0:58:35	2:09:47	4:32:28
0:28:10	0:58:56	2:10:33	4:34:06
0:28:20	0:59:17	2:11:20	4:35:43
0:28:30	0:59:38	2:12:06	4:37:20
0:28:40	0:59:59	2:12:52	4:38:58
0:28:50	1:00:20	2:13:39	4:40:35
0:29:00	1:00:40	2:14:25	4:42:12
0:29:10	1:01:01	2:15:11	4:43:50
0:29:20	1:01:22	2:15:58	4:45:27
0:29:30	1:01:43	2:16:44	4:47:04
0:29:40	1:02:04	2:17:30	4:48:41
0:29:50	1:02:25	2:18:17	4:50:19
0:30:00	1:02:46	2:19:03	4:51:56
0:30:10	1:03:07	2:19:49	4:53:33
0:30:20	1:03:28	2:20:36	4:55:11
0:30:30	1:03:49	2:21:22	4:56:48
0:30:40	1:04:10	2:22:09	4:58:25
0:30:50	1:04:31	2:22:55	5:00:03
0:31:00	1:04:52	2:23:41	5:01:40
0:31:10	1:05:12	2:24:28	5:03:17
0:31:20	1:05:33	2:25:14	5:04:55
0:31:30	1:05:54	2:26:00	5:06:32
0:31:40	1:06:15	2:26:47	5:08:09
0:31:50	1:06:36	2:27:33	5:09:47
0:32:00	1:06:57	2:28:19	5:11:24
0:32:10	1:07:18	2:29:06	5:13:01
0:32:20	1:07:39	2:29:52	5:14:38
0:32:30	1:08:00	2:30:38	5:16:16
0:32:40	1:08:21	2:31:25	5:17:53
0:32:50	1:08:42	2:32:11	5:19:30
0:33:00	1:09:03	2:32:57	5:21:08
0:33:10	1:09:23	2:33:44	5:22:45
0:33:20	1:09:44	2:34:30	5:24:22

5K	10K	HALF-MARATHON	MARATHON
0:33:30	1:10:05	2:35:16	5:26:00
0:33:40	1:10:26	2:36:03	5:27:37
0:33:50	1:10:47	2:36:49	5:29:14
0:34:00	1:11:08	2:37:36	5:30:52
0:34:10	1:11:29	2:38:22	5:32:29
0:34:20	1:11:50	2:39:08	5:34:06
0:34:30	1:12:11	2:39:55	5:35:44
0:34:40	1:12:32	2:40:41	5:37:21
0:34:50	1:12:53	2:41:27	5:38:58
0:35:00	1:13:14	2:42:14	5:40:35
0:35:10	1:13:35	2:43:00	5:42:13
0:35:20	1:13:55	2:43:46	5:43:50
0:35:30	1:14:16	2:44:33	5:45:27
0:35:40	1:14:37	2:45:19	5:47:05
0:35:50	1:14:58	2:46:05	5:48:42
0:36:00	1:15:19	2:46:52	5:50:19
0:36:10	1:15:40	2:47:38	5:51:57
0:36:20	1:16:01	2:48:24	5:53:34
0:36:30	1:16:22	2:49:11	5:55:11
0:36:40	1:16:43	2:49:57	5:56:49
0:36:50	1:17:04	2:50:43	5:58:26
0:37:00	1:17:25	2:51:30	6:00:03
0:37:10	1:17:46	2:52:16	6:01:41
0:37:20	1:18:07	2:53:03	6:03:18
0:37:30	1:18:27	2:53:49	6:04:55
0:37:40	1:18:48	2:54:35	6:06:32
0:37:50	1:19:09	2:55:22	6:08:10
0:38:00	1:19:30	2:56:08	6:09:47
0:38:10	1:19:51	2:56:54	6:11:24
0:38:20	1:20:12	2:57:41	6:13:02
0:38:30	1:20:33	2:58:27	6:14:39
0:38:40	1:20:54	2:59:13	6:16:16
0:38:50	1:21:15	3:00:00	6:17:54
0:39:00	1:21:36	3:00:46	6:19:31
0:39:10	1:21:57	3:01:32	6:21:08
0:39:20	1:22:18	3:02:19	6:22:46
0:39:30	1:22:39	3:03:05	6:24:23
0:39:40	1:22:59	3:03:51	6:26:00
0:39:50	1:23:20	3:04:38	6:27:37
0:40:00	1:23:41	3:05:24	6:29:15

REAL RUNNER REPORT

Dear all,

I wish to congratulate you on your great training plans. I have read your book *Run Less, Run Faster* and was convinced that this is the thing I was looking for. For years, I have failed to run a marathon below 3 hours since my first attempt in Berlin 2004 (3:02:11) until my last in Hamburg in April 2008 (3:00:59). I have started training with your plans 5 weeks ago and must admit that the key runs are harder than everything I did before, but I feel more relaxed overall, mainly by replacing junk miles with cycling. I feel improvements week after week and I am really looking forward to the target race (Essen Marathon) this spring. I will keep you guys posted on the result, of course! Anyway, when asked for a club I am running for I always fill in FIRST now.

Thanks a lot in advance,

Yours sincerely,

Dr. Thomas Alder
Operations General Manager, Biolitec
Bonn, Germany

FOLLOW-UP MESSAGE:

Bill, Scott –

I am pleased to inform you that I have finished the Essen Marathon in 2:58 on Sunday thanks to your great training schedules. This was my fifth try to break through the 3:00 wall having worked with different programs since the Berlin Marathon in 2004. As I avoided to take any risk to not finish in sub-3 but keeping my heart rate low, I am strongly convinced that I could have finished in an even faster time (my average heart rate during the race was 156).

CHAPTER 3

FIRST STEPS FOR THE NEW RUNNER

Can the FIRST program be used by the nonrunner? Absolutely. As long as you don't try to run too often, too long or too fast, too soon. We want new runners to enjoy their activity and keep enjoying it for a long time. That requires progressing slowly and not becoming a running dropout because of burnout, overtraining, or injury.

Injury, in particular, is common among novices because they are motivated and excited to go farther and faster. That zeal is reinforced because the gains as you begin an exercise program are significant. Those big gains encourage you to do more and more. We point out to beginners that small gains that seem subtle from day to day become dramatic over several months and years. We encourage all new runners to develop a solid base before tackling lofty goals, such as marathons. Use this book to help pace yourself.

We regularly hear from new runners who have never run a race of any distance; they often ask whether we have a marathon schedule for the new runner. Frequently, the person who contacts us is hoping to run a marathon in the next 6 months. While it is possible to survive the marathon distance by walking and running, we advise against attempting such a challenge without adequate preparation. Think 5K or 10K. It is much more enjoyable and healthier to train properly and still satisfy some reasonable intermediate goals prior to attempting the challenge of 26.2 miles.

In this chapter, you will find beginning runner training programs that progress conservatively, starting with a combination of walking and running. Follow the programs as designed, even if it feels too easy at first. Your body needs to adapt to the new stresses associated with running. Even if your cardiorespiratory system is not being stressed, the anatomical structures may be overtaxed and weakened due to your newfound activity. Gradually building a solid base from which to progress will ensure safe training and positive movement toward your goals.

At some point, your progress may become interrupted from fatigue. Pay attention to your body and recognize the signs of prolonged fatigue. Individuals vary considerably in how much training they can tolerate. Know your threshold of training. Insert a rest and recovery day regularly to prevent an overtrained condition. Sometimes it takes more than a day—it might take a very easy training week.

Many who decide to start running do so for weight loss. Be careful if you are overweight, because running is a weight-bearing activity and extra pounds add stress to the joints, muscles, bones, and connective tissue. Non-weight-bearing cross-training is especially valuable for losing weight without elevating your risk of injury.

BECOMING A RUNNER: THE FIRST STEPS

- Commit to a 5K race 3 months in advance.

- Schedule your workouts in advance.

- Get proper shoes.

- Get a training partner.

- Make training a habit.

- Cross-train (see Chapter 6).

- Do the FIRST stretches, drills, and strength training (see Chapters 12 and 13).

A COACH'S REPORT

Frankie Painter, a personal trainer in Deland, Florida, shared with us her success using the FIRST Novice 5K Program with her clients. Frankie reported that she has a 100 percent success rate with getting beginning runners to complete a 5K in 12 weeks following the Training Program in Table 3.1. She said that "no one has ever tried it and not liked it." Frankie said the fact that the program is based on time and not speed is very important to them. In addition to following the Novice Program, she stresses the importance of the stretches and strength exercises found in Chapters 12 and 13. She reported that some of her clients progressed to the Intermediate Program in Table 3.2 and the even more advanced program in Table 5.1. Following below is a report that Frankie forwarded to FIRST from one of her clients, Donna Nassick.

For years I watched runners as they ran; through my neighborhood, on the beach, or through the park. They all made it look so easy. Oh, how I wished that I had that sort of determination, discipline, and stamina. I tried once or twice. Got up in the morning deciding to give it a try . . . how hard could it be? I would run for as long as I could. Then practically collapse with my heart feeling like it would pop out of my chest. I just knew I would never be a runner.

Then one day I heard about a run/walk program that was being offered, with the goal being a 5K. I put the thought of it aside. How could I possibly start to run? After all, I was now 48 years old! But my interest was piqued. I went to the information session to see what it was all about. The trainer, Frankie, made us believe that it was possible with the FIRST run/walk program, so I signed up.

After the first couple of weeks I could not believe I was running a half a mile . . . without stopping!!! Then the half-mile turned into a mile, then 2 miles. How did running such short distances in the beginning turn into miles? As the weeks went by and I got closer to my goal I knew that there was no other way that I could have accomplished it without the run/walk program and the motivation from my trainer. I am thankful for both.

I did run my goal race, 3.1 miles, without stopping! You would have thought I had run a marathon!! I was that happy!!

BECOMING A RUNNER: Q AND A

Q. How do I get started?

A. First, make sure that you don't have any health problems that would prevent your starting an exercise program. If you have any existing medical problems or if you are over 40 years of age, we recommend that you get clearance to begin an exercise program from your physician.

Q. What about shoes?

A. Get proper shoes and clothing for exercise. There are many good running shoes available, each with different features. Find someone who is knowledgeable about running shoes to assist you in choosing a shoe that fits you properly. Try visiting several running specialty stores and seek advice from the knowledgeable sales assistants. It will take only two or three visits before you see trends in recommendations.

Q. When and where should I run?

A. Whether you run in the morning, at noon, or in the evening is largely a personal preference. Be realistic in deciding what regular schedule you are most likely to follow consistently. You don't have to work out at the same time each day. Plan ahead and consider your other obligations. Schedule a time for your run and consider it a priority. Consistency is essential in establishing a habit.

Choose a place that is safe to run. A track is a good place to start. Preferably, run in daylight. If you must run in the dark, choose a place that is well lit. You must be mindful of safety and security. Many runners have sprained an ankle stepping off the curb in the dark. It may be a good idea to invest in some reflective gear while you're at the running specialty store.

Q. How much should I do at first?

A. The FIRST program has three 12-week schedules that progress very gradually. Follow these schedules carefully and you will enjoy the benefits of improved fitness and health, along with the exhilaration of completing a 5K race. It's important that you don't try to do too much too soon. It's equally as important that you are faithful to the program and establish consistency in your training.

If you have done some running in your past or you regularly play other sports—basketball, tennis, cycling, etc.—and are not overweight, you may be able to begin with the intermediate program (Table 3.2) rather than the novice program (Table 3.1). The novice program is for someone who has been inactive and is just beginning to exercise.

Q. What if I am overweight?

A. The FIRST program is not a weight management program. However, regular physical activity expends energy and can assist you in weight loss. You must also be mindful that excess weight can be stressful to your joints and connective tissue. Combining a sensible diet with exercise is the safest and most effective way to reach a healthier weight.

If you are more than 30 pounds overweight, walking rather than running is advisable until you have reduced your excess weight. To help reduce stress on your joints, cross-training on non-weight-bearing exercise machines is also recommended until you have reduced your excess weight.

Q. Should I get a partner to train with or join a group?

A. *Yes!* Research shows clearly that those who train with a partner or with a regular running group comply better with an exercise schedule. The commitment to others appears to be a powerful motivator.

Q. Why does FIRST recommend starting with a 5K? Many people are joining marathon training groups even though they have no running experience.

A. FIRST believes that you need to establish a solid fitness base gradually before attempting a long race too soon; that can result in an injury. The exhilaration of running a 5K can be equal to or better than that of walking and running a longer race.

As health educators, we are interested in promoting running as a healthy, lifelong physical activity. Progressing gradually and developing the fitness and endurance for a 5K before moving on to a 10K, half-marathon, or marathon is a healthy approach. The physiological development for running peaks after about 8 to 10 years of training. Why not tackle these longer races when you are better prepared physically to do so?

You will have a much better running experience at these longer distances by running shorter races first. Many people join a charity training group without any running experience and complete the longer race—half-marathon or marathon—in survival mode. FIRST wants runners fully prepared for the race distance that they attempt.

Q: As a novice, can I use any of the rest of this manual?

A: Yes, once you complete the novice running program (Table 3.1) and complete your first 5K, then you can refer to the paces provided in the tables for the intermediate program (Table 3.2). After completing the intermediate training program, you will be ready to use the 5K training program (Table 5.1) found in Chapter 5.

Table 3.1

5K Novice Training Program

The program is designed to gradually move the inactive individual from walker to runner. It begins primarily with walking interspersed with short intervals of running during a half-hour workout. The first workout in Week #1 includes walking for 10 minutes. Following that 10 minutes of walking, you will run for 1 minute and then walk for 2 minutes, which will be repeated four times. After completing the fourth repetition of 1 minute of running, walk for 10 minutes to complete the workout. Run at a comfortable pace.

W=Walk **R**=Run

WEEK	WORKOUT #1	WORKOUT #2	WORKOUT #3
#1	W: 10 min (R: 1 min, W: 2 min) × 4 W: 10 min	W: 10 min (R: 1 min, W: 2 min) × 4 W: 10 min	W: 10 min (R: 1 min, W: 2 min) × 4 W: 10 min
#2	W: 10 min (R: 2 min, W: 2 min) × 3 W: 10 min	W: 10 min (R: 2 min, W: 2 min) × 3 W: 10 min	W: 10 min (R:2 min, W: 2 min) × 3 W: 10 min
#3	W: 10 min (R: 2 min, W: 1 min) × 4 W: 10 min	W: 10 min (R: 2 min, W: 1 min) × 4 W: 10 min	W: 10 min (R: 3 min, W: 2 min) × 3 W: 10 min
#4	W: 10 min (R: 3 min, W: 1 min) × 4 W: 10 min	W: 10 min (R: 3 min, W: 1 min) × 4 W: 10 min	W: 10 min (R: 3 min, W: 1 min) × 5 W: 10 min
#5	W: 10 min (R: 4 min, W: 2 min) × 4 W: 10 min	W: 10 min (R: 4 min, W: 2 min) × 4 W: 10 min	W: 10 min (R: 4 min, W: 1 min) × 5 W: 10 min
#6	W: 10 min (R: 4 min, W: 1 min) × 6 W: 10 min	W: 10 min (R: 4 min, W: 1 min) × 6 W: 10 min	W: 10 min (R: 5 min, W: 1 min) × 5 W: 10 min
#7	W: 10 min (R: 5 min, W: 1 min) × 6 W: 10 min	W: 10 min (R: 5 min, W: 1 min) × 6 W: 10 min	W: 10 min (R: 6 min, W: 1 min) × 5 W: 10 min
#8	W: 10 min R: 1 mile W: 5 min (R: 6 min, W: 1 min) × 3 W: 10 min	W: 10 min R: 1 mile W: 5 min (R: 6 min, W: 1 min) × 3 W: 10 min	W: 10 min R: 1 mile W: 5 min R: 1 mile W: 10 min
#9	W: 10 min R: 1.5 miles W: 10 min	W: 10 min R: 1.5 miles W: 5 min R: .5 mile W: 5 min	W: 10 min R: 2 miles W: 5 min
#10	W: 10 min R: 2 miles W: 5 min	W: 10 min R: 2 miles W: 5 min	W: 10 min R: 2.5 miles W: 5 min
#11	W: 10 min R: 2 miles W: 10 min	W: 10 min R: 2 miles W: 10 min	W: 10 min R: 3 miles W: 5 min
#12	W: 10 min R: 2 miles W: 10 min	W: 10 min R: 2 miles W: 10 min	W: 10 min R: 3.1 miles (5K) Race W: 5 min

Table 3.2

5K Intermediate Training Program

This training schedule is for the runner who has completed the novice training program or who can run 5 kilometers. The workouts include the basic FIRST key runs described in Chapter 5. The paces for the intermediate program can be found in Chapter 5 (Tables 5.6 and 5.7).

RI=Recovery Interval of 400 meter walk/jog after each repeat.

WEEK	KEY RUN #1	KEY RUN #2	KEY RUN #3
#1	10 min warmup run 2 × 400 (RI) 10 min cooldown run	1 mile warmup run 1 mile short tempo 1 mile cooldown run	3 miles @ mid-tempo pace
#2	10 min warmup run 3 × 400 (RI) 10 min cooldown run	1 mile warmup run 1 mile short tempo 1 mile cooldown run	3 miles @ mid-tempo pace
#3	10 min warmup run 4 × 400 (RI) 10 min cooldown run	1 mile warmup run 1 mile short tempo 1 mile cooldown run	3.5 miles @ mid-tempo pace
#4	10 min warmup run 2 × 400, 1 × 800 (RI) 10 min cooldown run	1 mile warmup run 1.5 mile short tempo 1 mile cooldown run	3.5 miles @ mid-tempo pace
#5	10 min warmup run 400, 600, 800 (RI) 10 min cooldown run	1 mile warmup run 1.5 mile short tempo 1 mile cooldown run	4 miles @ mid-tempo pace
#6	10 min warmup run 5 × 400 (RI) 10 min cooldown run	1 mile warmup run 1.5 mile short tempo 1 mile cooldown run	4 miles @ mid-tempo pace
#7	10 min warmup run 400, 2 × 800 (RI) 10 min cooldown run	1 mile warmup run 1.5 mile short tempo 1 mile cooldown run	4.5 miles @ mid-tempo pace
#8	10 min warmup run 2 × 1000 (RI) 10 min cooldown run	1 mile warmup run 2 mile short tempo 1 mile cooldown run	4.5 miles @ mid-tempo pace
#9	10 min warmup run 6 × 400 (RI) 10 min cooldown run	1 mile warmup run 2 mile short tempo 1 mile cooldown run	5 miles @ long tempo pace
#10	10 min warmup run 3 × 800 (RI) 10 min cooldown run	1 mile warmup run 2 mile short tempo 1 mile cooldown run	5 miles @ long tempo pace
#11	10 min warmup run 200, 400, 600, 800 (RI) 10 min cooldown run	1 mile warmup run 2 mile short tempo 1 mile cooldown run	5 miles @ long tempo pace
#12	10 min warmup run 4 × 400 (RI) 10 min cooldown run	2 miles easy 10 min walk	5K Race

Real Runner Report

I've been following your program for the last 2½ years—the total of my running career. I recently used the marathon plan to train for the Detroit Free Press Marathon a couple of weeks ago. I never would have thought that I could do five 20-mile runs AND train in the heat of summer, but I did. It was an exercise in mental toughness just as much as physical.

The stars aligned on race day—beautiful 50 degree weather, well-trained, well-rested, good hydration and fuel strategy in place, and no nagging injuries (which I attribute to my now regular yoga practice). My goal was a BQ time of 4:05. My first marathon, in January, was a mixed bag, but I had a time of 4:09, so I thought this was doable. My real goal—I have to admit—was to run sub-4:00. I had trained at paces based on a great half-marathon and 10K that I ran in the spring, and was targeting 8:50 pace.

The result? 3:53:34, never had a mile worse than 9:05, never felt as though I hit a "wall" (not the same as being fatigued, which I was!), and felt good afterwards. Bonus . . . I came in second in my age-group (it was a slow field)! My post-race week, I felt much better than my first marathon, and by Wednesday/Thursday I was ready to run again (which I didn't—took a break instead).

So the next day I joined the hordes online and am now officially registered to run Boston! This year has been a great running experience for me. Sub-2:00 half-marathon, sub-50 10K, and now Boston bound. I'm not sure I can top it for speed—but there are other goals out there.

So thanks from a happy customer and her dog-eared copy of your book.

Maura Gatowski
Beverly Hills, Michigan

REAL RUNNER REPORT

I heard about your program last fall and bought the book to train for Grandma's 2011 with the goal of qualifying for Boston 2012. I had run a half dozen marathons prior to using the FIRST training methods, with a PR of 3:13 when I was 28. I am 37 and have seven kids and a full-time job, so time for training is at a premium. The FIRST program really appealed to me from a time-management standpoint and diversity-in-activity perspective. I followed the program fairly closely and was generally able to run each session at the prescribed pace. Cross-trained on the bike, rowing machine, swimming, and cardio boot camps. No major injury setbacks during training and all systems were go last Saturday in Duluth. Race conditions were very favorable, but in the end, the training methods described in your book are what I believe helped propel me to a PR of 3:08 and a trip to Boston next year. Thanks for putting such a nice book together. It was a constant presence at my side throughout the months of training, and was a great resource for planning and tracking progress against the plan.

Regards,

Dennis Loperfido, CFA
Senior Investment Analyst
St. Paul, Minnesota

How to Follow the FIRST Training Program

CHAPTER 4

FIRST FUNDAMENTALS

To benefit fully from the FIRST **3plus2** training program you need to perform all five workouts each week. While the FIRST **3plus2** training program reduces the amount of running that you do weekly, it does not limit your training to 3 days per week. The total training volume includes three key running workouts and a minimum of two key cross-training workouts. The cumulative training effect of the workouts over 12 to 16 weeks translates into improved fitness, more speed, and better endurance. We have learned that most runners do not focus on speed and getting faster; their workouts lack variety; they do not allow for sufficient recovery; and they do not realize the value of cross-training.

We also hear from runners using our program that once they begin to follow a FIRST training schedule they find the paces challenging, but surprisingly meet those targets with serious efforts and proper recoveries. The FIRST training program is designed to gradually take runners toward more demanding workouts. The gradual progression of stress and overload stimulates improvement in the cardiorespiratory system and muscular tissue responsible for running performance.

In addition to the three key runs per week described in Chapter 5, an integral part of the **3plus2** Training Program is the aerobic cross-training.

The program includes a minimum of two cross-training workouts each week. In Chapter 6, there are descriptions of specific cross-training workouts that complement the three key running workouts. You may choose from among the different cross-training workouts those which you wish to use to supplement your running.

Is it possible to be fit and race successfully by completing the three key runs without doing the cross-training? By this point in the book, you should know that we believe strongly that cross-training is valuable and essential for optimal performance. However, we have reports of success—personal best times, Boston qualification—from runners who said that they did only the key run workouts. That being said, they likely would have run even faster had they included the cross-training in their weekly plan.

We recognize that most training books have chapters with comprehensive regimens for stretching, strength training, and form drills. In keeping with our philosophy of getting the optimal benefits from a minimal time commitment, we have selected what we consider the most beneficial and essential resistance training exercises (Chapter 12), stretches (Chapter 13), and running drills (Chapter 13) for you to include in your program. Once you become familiar with them, these 9 stretches and 11 strength training exercises will only take 30 minutes or less out of your day, three times each week, while the return on your time investment in terms of performance and reduced risk of injury is significant.

We, as runners, are well aware that stretching, strength training, and form drills are typically neglected. Runners assume that more time spent running will be more beneficial than devoting some of their limited time to these supplemental training exercises. Successful endurance performance is more than just running. If runners would devote just 5 to 10 percent of the time they spend running to these often overlooked, but important, aspects of their preparation, their running would improve.

Often, runners, in their zeal to get faster, engage in risky training that may not contribute to being healthier. Through repetition, many runners will incur overuse injuries and create muscular imbalances. We want to promote a fitter and healthier runner, just not a faster one. Smart training can help the runner be faster, fitter, and healthier. Chapters 5 and 6 provide the essentials of the FIRST training program designed to promote faster running, while contributing to one's overall health and prolonging one's running career. The information in the later chapters about stretching, strength training, form, year-round training, and nutrition are essential for becoming a well-balanced runner.

How to Start Using the Training Programs

All of the training target times and paces for all of the key runs in the next chapter are based on your current fitness level as represented by your most recent 5K race time or an estimate of your 5K race time. If you have a 5K race time that is representative of your current fitness level, use it for selecting your target times from Table 5.6 and for determining your mile or kilometer paces from Tables 5.7 and 5.8. If you do not have a 5K time that reflects your current fitness, but you have a recent 10K time that is indicative of your current fitness, go to Table 2.1 and find the 5K time equivalent to your 10K time and use it for selecting target times and paces from Tables 5.6–5.8.

If you do not have a 5K or 10K race finish time that represents your current fitness level, go to a 400-meter track and run 3 × 1600 meters (four laps around the track) with 1-minute recovery between each 1600 meters. During the 1-minute recovery, you can walk, but don't jog. Try to run the fastest time that you can maintain for all three 1600 meters. The goal is to have little variation in the times for the three 1600s. After you have finished, average the time of the three 1600 repeats and add 15 seconds to the average for a prediction of your 5K per-mile race pace. For example, if your average 1600-meter time is 7:20, add 15 seconds and use 7:35/mile as your predicted 5K race pace.

To find your metric equivalent, multiply your average 1600-meter time by .62 and add 9 seconds. For example, if your average 1600-meter time is 7:20, or 440 seconds, multiply by .62, which equals 272.8 seconds, or 4:32.8. Add 9 seconds and use 4:41.8, or 4:42/kilometer as your predicted 5K race pace.

Now that you have your 5K race pace, as calculated above, go to the pace tables in Appendix D and find your predicted 5K time of 23:34. You will use that 5K time for selecting your training target times and paces for the three Key Runs in Chapter 5.

If you do not have a 5K or 10K race finish time that represents your current fitness level and you do not do any speedwork—you do only distance running and you never run fast quarter-miles, half-miles, or miles—don't attempt to do the 3 × 1600-meter workout to determine your predicted 5K race time until you experience some speed training over the next 2 weeks.

In week one, go to the track and do 4 × 800 meters with a 400-meter jog in between 800 repeats. Try to run a pace that you can maintain throughout the four-repeat workout. Check your times for each repeat. The purpose of this workout is to accustom you to running faster than you normally run and to get a sense of pace for eventually performing the 3 × 1600-meter workout described in the previous section.

In the next week, go to the track and run 1 × 800 meters followed by a 400-meter jog recovery, followed by 1 × 1600 meters with a 400-meter jog recovery, and finish the workout with another 800 meters. Again, you should try to hold an even pace throughout the workout and record your times. That way, you'll have a sense of what you can maintain during the next week when you perform the 3 × 1600-meter workout to get your 5K predicted race time. You'll use it to select your training target times and paces from Tables 5.6–5.8.

In the first edition of this book, we indicated that you could use your half-marathon or marathon race finish times to predict your 5K race time by using Table 2.1. We found this approach is not a good predictor for many runners because it has become increasingly common for runners to race only half-marathons and marathons. Often they do no speed training and their training is limited to long, slow runs. For that reason, their predicted 5K race time using Table 2.1 would not be a valid predictor of their 5K race performance. Simply, they have focused only on endurance and not on speed. Therefore, if you have raced only half-marathons and marathons and have not included speed training—track repeats/interval training—you need to follow the instructions above to determine your current 5K fitness level.

Why is having a current, valid 5K race time important? The FIRST three key runs all specify a target time or pace for each run workout. To get the full benefits from each workout, you need to train at the appropriate intensity for producing a physiological adaptation that improves your fitness. Thousands of runners have reported that the training targets based on their 5K race times remarkably match their abilities. The common phrase reported in their messages to us is that the training targets are "challenging, but doable." Once you determine the 5K race time that represents your current fitness status, go to Chapter 5 and read about the three key runs.

Here is an example of a **3plus2** training week. It can be modified as long as the key runs are not performed on consecutive days. Chapter 5 describes in detail the three key runs and Chapter 6, the cross-training workouts.

The 3plus2 Training Week

DAY 1	DAY 2	DAY 3	DAY 4	DAY 5	DAY 6	DAY 7
Cross-Train #1	Key Run #1	Cross-Train #2	Key Run #2	Off	Key Run #3	Cross-Train or Rest

Day 1 Cross-Training Workout #1 (For 5K and 10K training, see Tables 6.1 and 6.2; for half-marathon and marathon training, see Tables 6.3 and 6.4.)

Day 2 Key Run #1: Track Repeats (See Tables 5.1–5.5 for training schedules and Table 5.6 for training target times.)

Day 3 Cross-Training Workout #2 (For 5K and 10K training, see Tables 6.1 and 6.2, for half-marathon and marathon training, see Tables 6.3 and 6.4.)

Day 4 Key Run #2: Tempo Run (See Tables 5.1–5.5 for training schedules and Table 5.7 for paces.)

Day 5 Rest Day

Day 6 Key Run #3: Long Run (See Tables 5.1–5.5 for training schedules and Table 5.8 for paces.)

Day 7 Rest Day or Optional Cross-Training

TRAINING SUMMARY FOR 5K, 10K, HALF-MARATHON AND MARATHON

Training for a 5K: Complete three key runs from Table 5.1 and two cross-training workouts from Tables 6.1 and 6.2. Paces for the key runs are in Tables 5.6–5.8.

Training for a 10K: Complete three key runs from Table 5.2 and two cross-training workouts from Tables 6.1 and 6.2. Paces for the key runs are in Tables 5.6–5.8.

Training for a Half-Marathon: Complete three key runs from Table 5.3 and two cross-training workouts from Tables 6.3 and 6.4. Paces for the key runs are in Tables 5.6–5.8.

Training for a Marathon: Complete three key runs from either Table 5.4 or 5.5 and two cross-training workouts from Tables 6.3 and 6.4. Paces for the key runs are in Tables 5.6–5.8.

REAL RUNNER REPORT

Dear FIRST,

After being an on-off runner for several years, I took a more serious approach 2 years ago and completed some half-marathons in the 2:30 range. Then I succumbed to peer pressure and tried my first full marathon, managing it in 5:08, though this attempt left me with a painful calf injury.

In hindsight, I realized that I had ramped up too soon, and I decided to re-evaluate my running goals. The fact is that in India, running is still in its infancy, and the general perception is that to improve your timing, you have to run more. But this seemed to me to be a recipe for disaster—increased likelihood of injuries due to tired muscles, mental and physical fatigue from excessive running, as well as a strain on managing my other responsibilities in life.

My inner voice told me to settle on a strong half before looking at the full again. It didn't help that I also had limited time given that I had just changed to a more demanding job.

Around this time, a fellow runner introduced me to your book, *Run Less. Run Faster,* and it seemed to be the perfect answer for my next half-marathon later this year. As a systematic person, I am approaching my training very seriously, maintaining a precise log of each run with power yoga, swimming, and strength training serving as the stipulated cross training.

What especially impresses me is that each run needs to be purposeful. I like that each training run has a mileage and pace target calculated based on my best 5K time. Yes, the initial weeks were difficult, and I particularly struggled with the interval repeats. But I can sense a change in my running as my body adapts o the progressive stress, and, with the intermittent rest days from running, I come back hungry to run.

The results are amazing. Earlier, my best half marathon pace was 6:16 min/K, but just 8 weeks into the FIRST program, I am running at a tempo pace of 5:11 and long run pace of 5:28. I am also relatively injury-free now.

My goal using your FIRST program is to finish my next half-marathon under 2 hours. And, given that on a recent long 20K training run I clocked 1:49, I feel very confident of achieving my immediate running goal. And this will give me that essential mental strength to target yet more aggressive timings in the years ahead.

I am sure you get many such letters, but possibly I am the first writer from India. But the running space here is growing fast and I am sure that your FIRST program will find many takers here soon, as the results speak for themselves.

Ms. Vaishali Kasture
Senior Corporate
Bangalore, India

REAL RUNNER REPORT

Dear Sirs,

I wrote you a message about 3 years ago when I finished my second marathon in 2:59, having trained according to your great program. (First marathon, I did 3:18 in 2007—following a different plan with five to six runs per week. By training so much I got a shin split and the doc told me that I'd either have to undergo surgery or reduce my mileage. That's how I came across your concept.)

I just wanted to let you know that I'm more than happy: I continued to do a few races per year (two 10Ks, one half-marathon), always training according to the FIRST principle. Last Sunday I did my third marathon (Berlin) after a 3-year break and I enjoyed myself while finishing in 2:49:12—at the age of 41!

It's just unbelievable. About every amateur runner I know keeps telling me that you can't run under 3 hours with only three runs per week. I'm really looking forward to what these guys will tell me now.

For me it's the perfect match—that's for sure. So thanks again for sharing these great training insights—you made a really happy man out of me!

Daniel Lipp
Senior Software Developer
Rheinfelden, Germany

CHAPTER 5

THREE QUALITY RUNS

The "3" of the **3plus2** Training Program

"I was skeptical when I started your training program, but I found that the challenging, but doable, three key run workouts caused me to get stronger and faster week after week." That's the most common refrain from readers who adhere to the FIRST training programs. The three-runs-per-week schedule defies conventional thinking about the necessity of piling on the miles.

Most runners who incorporate the three quality runs find that their fitness improves as do their race times. What explains this? Most runners focus on the frequency and duration of their training. Their conversations begin with "How many times did you run" and end with "How many miles did you log this week?" They neglect the importance of *intensity*—the pace of each workout. Try running the paces designated in the tables provided in this chapter and watch your race times improve.

While a certain fitness base is necessary, quality performances are determined more by intensity than by volume. Workouts that cause you to go really hard, recover, and go hard again have significant physiological benefits. Workouts sustained at a moderately hard effort for 20 to 30 minutes also train your body to exercise for long periods near your maximum effort. Doing long runs at speeds progressively closer to your marathon pace causes you to adapt to the stress of running hard for several hours to prepare for a marathon.

This chapter supplies you with the training paces appropriate for your current fitness level—paces that will lead to improvements in your fitness level and future running performances. It also provides the nuts-and-bolts descriptions for your three quality runs per week, the heart of the **3plus2** training program. You will find all of the details necessary for performing the three weekly quality runs. Following the breakdown of the overall design of the program are tables that show you how to determine your target time and pace for each run (see Tables 5.6–5.8) and the training schedules for 5K, 10K, half-marathon and marathon races (see Tables 5.1–5.5). First, however, we present a brief discussion of the science underlying the FIRST program.

THREE QUALITY RUNS: THE SCIENCE

The theoretical concept underlying the FIRST training regimen is that each run be performed with a goal of improving one of the primary physiological processes and running performance variables. The training programs are designed to help runners train effectively and efficiently while avoiding overtraining and injury.

Maximal oxygen consumption (VO$_2$ max) is a measure of the ability of an athlete to produce energy aerobically. One might say that maximal oxygen consumption gives a runner an idea of how large an engine he or she has to work with. Normally, a higher VO$_2$ max indicates more work can be performed during a given time period. This simply means that an individual with a higher VO$_2$ max should be able to run faster than an otherwise comparable runner with a lower VO$_2$ max. A high maximal capacity to deliver oxygenated blood means there is the potential for more muscles to be active simultaneously during exercise. Values for VO$_2$ max typically range between 40 and 80 milliliters of oxygen per kilogram of body weight. Research has shown VO_2 max to increase as much as 20 percent through a combination of endurance and interval training. VO_2 max and submaximal exercise capacity are limited by different mechanisms. VO_2 max appears to be related more to cardiovascular factors, such as maximal cardiac output, whereas skeletal muscle metabolic factors, including respiratory enzyme activity, play more of a role in determining submaximal exercise capacity.

Lactate threshold (LT) is a measure of metabolic fitness. Lactate is an organic by-product of anaerobic metabolism, and its accumulation in the blood is used to evaluate the intensity that a runner can maintain for extended periods of time—usually 30 minutes or more. Lactate threshold and maximal steady state lactate levels are indications of how well one's muscles are trained to do endurance-type work. Most people, except the most highly trained athletes, are limited by metabolic fitness rather than cardiovascular fitness. Highly trained endurance athletes become "centrally limited," meaning they can work at extreme heart rates without severe muscle fatigue. An untrained individual might reach LT at about 50 to 60 percent of his or her maximum heart rate, whereas a well-trained runner won't reach lactate threshold until about 80 to 95 percent of his or her maximum heart rate.

Running economy is the amount of oxygen being consumed relative to the runner's body weight and the speed at which the runner is traveling. Unnecessary body motion results in an increase in oxygen consumption and thus a decrease in running economy. Running economy can be expressed either as the velocity achieved for a given rate of oxygen consumption or the VO_2 needed to maintain a given running speed. Running at a given submaximal pace and using less oxygen indicate that a runner is more economical or has improved his or her running economy. This determinant of running performance generally takes the longest period of training for measurable improvements.

Training at the appropriate intensity is generally recognized as the most important factor for improving each of the three elements. For that reason, each workout needs to have the appropriate intensity, or running pace, that stimulates the physiological adaptation needed for improving.

THREE QUALITY RUNS: THE ESSENTIALS

Types of Training

ELEMENTS	KEY RUN #1: TRACK REPEATS	KEY RUN #2: TEMPO RUN	KEY RUN #3: LONG RUN
Purpose	Improve VO$_2$ max running speed, and running economy	Improve endurance by raising lactate threshold	Improve endurance by raising aerobic metabolism
Intensity	5K race pace or slightly faster	Comfortably hard; 15 to 45 sec slower than 5K race pace	Approximately 30 sec slower than goal marathon pace
Duration of Each Run	10 minutes or less	20 to 45 min at tempo pace	60 to 180 min
Frequency	Repeat shorter segments until quality work totals about 5K per session	One tempo run per week	One long run per week

KEY RUN #1: TRACK REPEATS

Warmup

Warm up for 10 to 20 minutes of easy jogging followed by four 100-meter strides. Completion of the strides will make the initial track repeats much easier and reduce the shock of going from an easy warmup jog to a near all-out effort on the repeats. Stay comfortable with the strides and focus on good form. You shouldn't be straining during the strides. Gradually accelerate for 80 meters until you reach approximately 90 percent of full speed, and then decelerate over the final 20 meters. Recover for 30 seconds or less and repeat.

In Chapter 13, two key drills that will help your form are described and illustrated on pages 179–182. These two key drills can be incorporated into your warmup strides. After completing two 100-meter strides, begin the third 100 meters by doing butt kicks for 20 meters and then gradually accelerating for 60 meters and decelerate for 20 meters. Recover for 30 seconds, begin the next 100 meters, and do high knee lifts for 20 meters, and then gradually accelerate for 60 meters and decelerate for 20 meters.

The Track Repeats

The track repeats include running relatively short distances of 400 meters to 2000 meters, interspersed with brief recovery intervals on a repeated basis. Track repeats are designed to improve maximal oxygen consumption, running economy, and speed. Most of these workouts total about 5000 meters of fast running per session. Including warmup and cooldown, Key Run #1 typically totals 5 to 6 miles or 8 to 10 kilometers.

Caution: Most runners can run the first few repeats faster than the specified target time. However, the challenge is to run the entire workout at the target time with little or no deviation in the times for each repeat. Also, the objective is not to run the repeats as fast as you can; you have two other key runs to perform for the week. Do not sacrifice meeting the target times for the tempo and long runs by running the repeats at an exhausting speed that does not provide sufficient recovery for Key Runs # 2 and #3.

Cooldown

After a challenging workout of repeats on the track, a cooldown is important. Jog slowly for 10 to 15 minutes.

Track Repeat Example 1: 6 × 800 (90 sec RI)

Repeat an 800-meter run six times, with a recovery interval (RI) of 90 seconds. In between the repeats, you recover by walking/jogging for 90 seconds. After the 90 seconds of recovery, you will start the next 800-meter run. You run all of the 800 meters at the same prescribed target time, which is found in Table 5.6. The goal of the workout is to keep a small range of times for the 800 meters. For example, rather than a set like 3:00, 2:58, 3:04, 3:08, 3:09, 3:02, shoot for a more consistent range of times, such as 3:02, 3:01, 3:02, 3:02, 3:03, 3:02. There should not be more than a couple of seconds' difference in your times for the repeats.

Track Repeat Example 2: 5 × 1000 (400m RI)

Repeat runs of 1000 meters (2.5 times around a 400-meter track) five times with a 400-meter walk/jog as a recovery between repeat runs. Using your prescribed training pace for 1000 meters, try running the first repeat at the target time (found in Table 5.6). Check your time after finishing the first repeat to make sure you aren't running too fast or too slowly. Jog 400 meters at a comfortable pace for your recovery (for most people, this lap will take 2 to 4 minutes). At the end of the jog recovery, begin the second repeat, concentrating on maintaining the prescribed pace. The times for running the five 1000-meter repeats should vary no more than a few seconds.

The FIRST training program emphasizes the importance of keeping a very small range of times for the entire workout. The target paces should be realistic and challenging, but not so difficult that you are unable to recover for Key Run #2. Our emphasis that the entire set of repeats be run within a range of only a couple of seconds pretty much ensures that you won't overdo it.

KEY RUN #2: TEMPO RUN

Warmup

Tempo runs begin with easy running for 1 or 2 miles prior to the faster tempo phase of the workout. As with the strides on the track, the pace should gradually increase during the easy miles, so that you are close to tempo pace by the end of the warmup.

The Tempo Run

The tempo portion of the workout is typically 3 to 5 miles at 10K pace or slightly slower. For marathon training, the tempo portion is extended to 8 to 10 miles at planned marathon pace.

Cooldown

A mile or 10 minutes of easy running is recommended for a cooldown after the tempo phase of the run.

Example: 1 mile warmup, 2 miles at ST and 1 mile cooldown

Start slowly and gradually pick up the pace, and after 1 mile, run the next 2 miles at the designated pace based on your 5K race pace (see Table 5.7). This short-tempo pace (ST) is approximately 15 seconds slower than your per-mile 5K race pace and 9 seconds slower than your per-kilometer pace. After the 2-mile tempo run, slow down and run an easy cooldown mile. In this example, Key Run #2 is a continuous 4-mile run.

Key Run #3: Long Run

Warmup

While there is not a specific warmup for your long run, the early part of the long run can serve as the warmup. The recommended long run pace need not be achieved during the first couple of miles or kilometers.

The Long Run

The long run (relative to your goals and present training mileage) requires steady running from 6 to 20 miles at a pace equal to one's 5K pace plus 45 seconds for the 5K and 10K long runs. For the half-marathon and marathon long runs, the long run pace is equal to one's 5K pace plus 75 to 90 seconds, or 15 to 30 seconds per mile or 9 to 19 seconds per kilometer slower than planned marathon pace.

Try starting your training runs a bit slower than the prescribed pace and then pick up the pace in the middle section of your training run. Try to have a strong finish over the last couple of miles (kilometers) of your long training runs. If you run faster than recommended pace during the middle phase of the long run, it can offset the earlier slower pace so you can meet the average targeted pace for the entire run.

Cooldown

Ten minutes of easy walking after a long run serves as a good cooldown. Drinking a sports drink or recovery drink during these 10 minutes will aid your recovery (see Chapter 7). Doing some of the basic static stretches described in Chapter 13 is valuable.

Example: 15 miles at MP + 30

Run 15 miles, 30 seconds per mile slower than planned marathon pace. For a runner with a target marathon time of 3:10, or 7:15/mile pace, this long run might begin with a 7:55 mile followed by a 7:40 mile before settling into a 7:45/mile pace. After 5 miles of running at a 7:45/mile pace, you may want to try the next 3 or 4 miles at 7:35-40 pace before running the last few miles at a 7:45/mile pace. Or you may want to hold the 7:45/mile pace up through 12 miles and then try to run the last 3 miles faster. You can alternate strategies from one long training run to the next. The metric version of this workout is 24K at MP + 19. Run 24 kilometers 19 seconds per kilometer slower than planned marathon pace. For a runner with a target marathon time of 3:10 or 4:30/kilometer pace, this long run might begin with a 4:55 pace followed by a 4:45 kilometer before settling into a 4:49/kilometer pace. After 8 kilometers of running at a 4:49/kilometer pace, you may want to try the next 5 to 7 kilometers at a 4:40 to 4:45 pace before running the last few kilometers at a 4:49/kilometer pace. Or you may want to hold the 4:49/kilometer pace up through 20K and then try to run the last 4K faster.

Detailed Training Schedules for Four Popular Race Distances and Training Paces

FIRST's three key run schedules for distances of 5K, 10K, half-marathon, and marathon follow in Tables 5.1 through 5.5. To find the appropriate training target time or pace for a specific distance, refer to Tables 5.6 to 5.8. If you have not run a recent 5K, refer to the instructions on page 45.

Table 5.1

5K Training Program: The Three Quality Runs

RI = Recovery Interval; which may be a timed recovery interval or a distance that you walk/jog.

Paces: **ST** = Short Tempo; **MT** = Mid-Tempo; **LT** = Long Tempo. See Table 5.7.

Key Run #1 (Track Repeats) begins with 10- to 20-minute warmup; ends with 10-minute cooldown. See Table 5.6 for target times.

Key Run #2 (Tempo Run) begins with 1-mile (1.5K) warmup; ends with 1-mile (1.5K) cooldown. See Table 5.7.

Metric equivalents appear in bold italics.

WEEK	KEY RUN #1 (TRACK REPEATS)	KEY RUN #2 (TEMPO RUN)	KEY RUN #3 (LONG RUN)
12	8 × 400 (400 RI)	2 miles *(3K)* at ST	5 miles *(8K)* at LT
11	5 × 800 (400 RI)	3 miles *(5K)* at ST	6 miles *(10K)* at LT
10	2 × 1600 (400 RI) 1 × 800 (400 RI)	2 miles *(3K)* at ST 1 mile *(1.5K)* easy 2 miles *(3K)* at ST	5 miles *(8K)* at LT
9	400, 600, 800, 800, 600, 400 (400 RI)	4 miles *(6.5K)* at MT	6 miles *(10K)* at LT
8	4 × 1000 (400 RI)	3 miles *(5K)* at ST	7 miles *(11K)* at LT
7	1600, 1200, 800, 400 (400 RI)	1 mile *(1.5K)* at ST 1 mile *(1.5K)* easy 1 mile *(1.5K)* at ST 1 mile *(1.5K)* easy 1 mile *(1.5K)* at ST	6 miles *(10K)* at LT
6	10 × 400 (90 sec RI)	4 miles *(6.5K)* at MT	8 miles *(13K)* at LT
5	6 × 800 (90 sec RI)	2 miles *(3K)* at ST 1 mile *(1.5K)* easy 2 miles *(3K)* at ST	7 miles *(11K)* at LT
4	4 × 1200 (400 RI)	3 miles *(5K)* at ST	7 miles *(11K)* at LT
3	5 × 1000 (400 RI)	2 miles *(3K)* at ST 1 mile *(1.5K)* easy 1 mile *(1.5K)* at ST 1 mile *(1.5K)* easy 2 miles *(3K)* at ST	7 miles *(11K)* at LT
2	3 × 1600 (400 RI)	3 miles *(5K)* at ST	6 miles *(10K)* at LT
1	6 × 400 (60 sec RI)	3 miles *(5K)* easy No additional warmup or cooldown	5K Race

Table 5.2

10K Training Program: The Three Quality Runs

RI = Recovery Interval; which may be a timed recovery interval or a distance that you walk/jog.
Paces: **ST** = Short Tempo; **MT** = Mid-Tempo; **LT** = Long Tempo. See Table 5.7.
Key Run #1 (Track Repeats) begins with 10- to 20-minute warmup; ends with 10-minute cooldown. See Table 5.6 for target times.
Key Run #2 (Tempo Run) begins with 1-mile (1.5K) warmup; ends with 1-mile (1.5K) cooldown. See Table 5.7.
Metric equivalents appear in bold italics.

WEEK	KEY RUN #1 (TRACK REPEATS)	KEY RUN #2 (TEMPO RUN)	KEY RUN #3 (LONG RUN)
12	8 × 400 (400 RI)	3 miles *(5K)* at ST	6 miles *(10K)* at LT
11	5 × 800 (400 RI)	2 miles *(3K)* at ST 1 mile *(1.5K)* easy 2 miles *(3K)* at ST	7 miles *(11K)* at LT
10	2 × 1600 (400 RI); 1 × 800 (400 RI)	4 miles *(6.5K)* at MT	8 miles *(13K)* at LT
9	400, 600, 800, 800, 600, 400 (400 RI)	2 miles *(3K)* at ST 1 mile *(1.5K)* easy 1 mile *(1.5K)* at ST 1 mile *(1.5K)* easy 2 miles *(3K)* at ST	9 miles *(14K)* at LT
8	4 × 1000 (400 RI)	4 miles *(6.5K)* at ST	10 miles *(16K)* at LT
7	1600, 1200, 800, 400 (400 RI)	5 miles *(8K)* at MT	8 miles *(13K)* at LT
6	10 × 400 (90 sec RI)	3 miles *(6.5K)* at ST	10 miles *(16K)* at LT
5	6 × 800 (90 sec RI)	1 mile *(1.5K)* at ST 1 mile *(1.5K)* easy 2 miles *(3K)* at ST 1 mile *(1.5K)* easy 1 mile *(1.5K)* at ST	8 miles *(13K)* at LT
4	4 × 1200 (400 RI)	3 miles *(5K)* at ST	10 miles *(16K)* at LT
3	5 × 1000 (400 RI)	6 miles *(10K)* at MT	8 miles *(13K)* at LT
2	3 × 1600 (400 RI)	3 miles *(5K)* at ST	7 miles *(11K)* at LT
1	6 × 400 (60 sec RI)	3 miles *(5K)* easy No additional warmup or cooldown	10K Race

Table 5.3

Half-Marathon Training Program: The Three Quality Runs

RI = Recovery Interval; which may be a timed recovery interval or a distance that you walk/jog.
Paces: **HMP** = Half Marathon Pace; **ST** = Short Tempo; **MT** = Mid-Tempo, **LT** = Long Tempo. A plus sign (+) followed by a figure indicates seconds per mile or kilometer. See Tables 5.7–5.8.
Key Run #1 (Track Repeats) begins with 10- to 20-minute warmup; ends with 10-minute cooldown. See Table 5.6 for target times.
Metric equivalents appear in bold italics.

WEEK	KEY RUN #1 (TRACK REPEATS)	KEY RUN #2 (TEMPO RUN)	KEY RUN #3 (LONG RUN)
16	12 × 400 (90 sec RI)	2 miles *(3K)* easy 3 miles *(5K)* at ST 1 mile *(1.5K)* easy	8 miles at HMP + 20 *12.5K at HMP + 13*
15	400, 600, 800, 1200, 800, 600, 400 (400 RI)	1 mile *(1.5K)* easy 5 miles *(8K)* at MT 1 mile *(1.5K)* easy	9 miles at HMP + 20 *14K at HMP + 13*
14	6 × 800 (90 sec RI)	2 miles *(3K)* easy 3 miles *(5K)* at ST 1 mile *(1.5K)* easy	10 miles easy *16K easy*
13	5 × 1000 (400 RI)	1 mile *(1.5K)* easy 3 miles *(5K)* at ST 1 mile *(1.5K)* easy	9 miles at HMP + 20 *14K at HMP + 13*
12	3 × 1600 (60 sec RI)	1 mile *(1.5K)* easy 6 miles *(10K)* at LT 1 mile *(1.5K)* easy	11 miles at HMP + 30 *18K at HMP + 19*
11	2 × 1200 (2 min RI); 4 × 800 (2 min RI)	1 mile *(1.5K)* easy 2 miles *(3K)* at MT 1 mile *(1.5K)* easy 2 miles *(3K)* at MT 1 mile *(1.5K)* easy	10 miles at HMP + 20 *16K at HMP + 13*
10	6 × 800 (90 sec RI)	1 mile *(1.5K)* easy 5 miles *(8K)* at MT 1 mile *(1.5K)* easy	12 miles at HMP + 30 *19K at HMP + 19*
9	2 × (6 × 400) (90 sec RI); (2 min 30 sec RI between sets)	1 mile *(1.5K)* easy 2 miles *(3K)* at MT 1 mile *(1.5K)* easy 2 miles *(3K)* at MT 1 mile *(1.5K)* easy	8 miles at HMP + 20 *12.5K at HMP + 13*
8	2 × 1600 (60 sec RI); 2 × 800 (60 sec RI)	1 mile *(1.5K)* easy 5 miles *(8K)* at MT 1 mile *(1.5K)* easy	13 miles at HMP + 30 *21K at HMP + 19*
7	4 × 1200 (2 min RI)	1 mile *(1.5K)* easy 6 miles *(10K)* at MT 1 mile *(1.5K)* easy	10 miles at HMP + 20 *16K at HMP + 13*
6	1000, 2000, 1000, 1000 (400 RI)	1 mile *(1.5K)* easy 5 miles *(8K)* at MT 1 mile *(1.5K)* easy	14 miles at HMP + 30 *22K at HMP + 19*
5	3 × 1600 (400 RI)	6 miles *(10K)* easy	10 miles at HMP + 20 *16K at HMP + 13*

WEEK	KEY RUN #1 (TRACK REPEATS)	KEY RUN #2 (TEMPO RUN)	KEY RUN #3 (LONG RUN)
4	10 × 400 (400 RI)	1 mile *(1.5K)* easy 5 miles *(8K)* at MT 1 mile *(1.5K)* easy	15 miles at HMP + 30 *25K at HMP + 19*
3	2 × 1200 (2 min RI); 4 × 800 (2 min RI)	1 mile *(1.5K)* easy 5 miles *(8K)* at MT 1 mile *(1.5K)* easy	12 miles at HMP + 20 *19K at HMP + 13*
2	5 × 1000 (400 RI)	2 miles *(3K)* easy 3 miles *(5K)* at ST 1 mile *(1.5K)* easy	8 miles at HMP + 20 *12.5K at HMP + 13*
1	6 × 400 (400 RI)	3 miles *(5K)* easy No additional warmup or cooldown	Half-Marathon 13.1 miles *(21.1K)*

Table 5.4

Novice Marathon Training Program: The Three Quality Runs

RI = Recovery Interval; which may be a timed recovery interval or a distance that you walk/jog.
Paces: **HMP** = Half-Marathon Pace; **ST** = Short Tempo; **MT** = Mid-Tempo; **LT** = Long Tempo. A plus sign (+) followed by a figure indicates seconds per mile or kilometer. See Tables 5.7–5.8.
Key Run #1 (Track Repeats) begins with 10- to 20-minute warmup; ends with 10-minute cooldown. See Table 5.6 for target times.
Metric equivalents appear in bold italics.

WEEK	KEY RUN #1 (TRACK REPEATS)	KEY RUN #2 (TEMPO RUN)	KEY RUN #3 (LONG RUN)
16	3 × 1600 (400 RI)	2 miles *(3K)* easy 2 miles *(3K)* at ST 2 miles *(3K)* easy	8 miles at MP + 30 *13K at MP + 19*
15	4 × 800 (2 min RI)	1 mile *(1.5K)* easy 5 miles *(8K)* at MP 1 mile *(1.5K)* easy	9 miles at MP + 45 *15K at MP + 28*
14	1200, 1000, 800, 600, 400 (200 RI)	1 mile *(1.5K)* easy 5 miles *(8K)* at LT 1 mile *(1.5K)* easy	10 miles at MP + 45 *16K at MP + 28*
13	5 × 1000 (400 RI)	1 mile *(1.5K)* easy 4 miles *(6.5K)* at MT 1 mile *(1.5K)* easy	11 miles at MP + 45 *17K at MP + 28*
12	3 × 1600 (400 RI)	2 miles *(3K)* easy 3 miles *(5K)* at ST 1 mile *(1.5K)* easy	12 miles at MP + 45 *20K at MP + 28*
11	2 × 1200 (2 min RI); 4 × 800 (2 min RI)	1 mile *(1.5K)* easy 5 miles *(8K)* at MT 1 mile *(1.5K)* easy	14 miles at MP + 45 *22K at MP + 28*

WEEK	KEY RUN #1 (TRACK REPEATS)	KEY RUN #2 (TEMPO RUN)	KEY RUN #3 (LONG RUN)
10	6 × 800 (90 sec RI)	1 mile *(1.5K)* easy 6 miles *(10K)* at LT 1 mile *(1.5K)* easy	10 miles at MP + 15 *16K at MP + 9*
9	2 × (6 × 400) (90 sec RI); (2 min 30 sec RI between sets)	2 miles *(3K)* easy 3 miles *(5K)* at ST 1 mile *(1.5K)* easy	15 miles at MP + 30 *24K at MP + 19*
8	2 × 1600 (60 sec RI); 2 × 800 (60 sec RI)	1 mile *(1.5K)* easy 4 miles *(6.5K)* at MT 1 mile *(1.5K)* easy	16 miles at MP + 30 *20K at MP + 19*
7	4 × 1200 (2 min RI)	10 miles *(16K)* at MP	12 miles at MP + 20 *24K at MP + 12*
6	1000, 2000, 1000, 1000 (400 RI)	1 mile *(1.5K)* easy 5 miles *(8K)* at MP 1 mile *(1.5K)* easy	18 miles at MP + 45 *30K at MP + 28*
5	3 × 1600 (400 RI)	10 miles *(16K)* at MP	13 miles at MP + 15 *21K at MP + 9*
4	10 × 400 (400 RI)	10-minute warmup 8 miles *(13K)* at MP 10-minute cooldown	20 miles at MP + 30 *32K at MP + 19*
3	8 × 800 (90 sec RI)	1 mile *(1.5K)* easy 5 miles *(8K)* at MT 1 mile *(1.5K)* easy	13 miles at MP *21K at MP*
2	5 × 1000 (400 RI)	2 miles *(3K)* easy 3 miles *(5K)* at ST 1 mile *(1.5K)* easy	8 miles at MP *13K at MP*
1	6 × 400 (400 RI)	10 min warmup 3 miles *(5K)* at MP 10 min cooldown	Marathon 26.2 miles *(42.2K)*

Table 5.5

Marathon Training Program:
The Three Quality Runs

RI = Recovery Interval; which may be a timed recovery interval or a distance that you walk/jog.
Paces: **HMP** = Half-Marathon Pace; **ST** = Short Tempo; **MT** = Mid-Tempo; **LT** = Long Tempo. A
plus sign (+) followed by a figure indicates seconds per mile or kilometer. See Tables 5.7–5.8.
Key Run #1 begins with 10- to 20-minute warmup; ends with 10-minute cooldown. See Table
5.6 for target times.
Metric equivalents appear in bold italics.

WEEK	KEY RUN #1 (TRACK REPEATS)	KEY RUN #2 (TEMPO RUN)	KEY RUN #3 (LONG RUN)
16	3 × 1600 (400 RI)	2 miles *(3K)* easy 2 miles *(3K)* at ST 2 miles *(3K)* easy	13 miles at MP + 30 ***21K at MP + 19***
15	4 × 800 (2 min RI)	1 mile *(1.5K)* easy 5 miles *(8K)* at MP 1 mile *(1.5K)* easy	15 miles at MP + 45 ***24K at MP + 28***
14	1200, 1000, 800, 600, 400 (200 RI)	1 mile *(1.5K)* easy 5 miles *(8K)* at LT 1 mile *(1.5K)* easy	17 miles at MP + 45 ***27K at MP + 28***
13	5 × 1000 (400 RI)	1 mile *(1.5K)* easy 4 miles *(6.5K)* at MT 1 mile *(1.5K)* easy	20 miles at MP + 60 ***32K at MP + 37***
12	3 × 1600 (400 RI)	2 miles *(3K)* easy 3 miles *(5K)* at ST 1 mile *(1.5K)* easy	18 miles at MP + 45 ***29K at MP + 28***
11	2 × 1200 (2 min RI); 4 × 800 (2 min RI)	1 mile *(1.5K)* easy 5 miles *(8K)* at MT 1 mile *(1.5K)* easy	20 miles at MP + 45 ***32K at MP + 28***
10	6 × 800 (90 sec RI)	1 mile *(1.5K)* easy 6 miles *(10K)* at LT 1 mile *(1.5K)* easy	13 miles at MP + 15 ***21K at MP + 9***
9	2 × (6 × 400) (90 sec RI) (2 min 30 sec RI between sets)	2 miles *(3K)* easy 3 miles *(5K)* at ST 1 mile *(1.5K)* easy	18 miles at MP + 30 ***29K at MP + 19***
8	2 × 1600 (60 sec RI); 2 × 800 (60 sec RI)	1 mile *(1.5K)* easy 4 miles *(6.5K)* at MT 1 mile *(1.5K)* easy	20 miles at MP + 30 ***32K at MP + 19***
7	4 × 1200 (2 min RI)	10 miles *(16K)* at MP	15 miles at MP + 20 ***24K at MP + 12***
6	1000, 2000, 1000, 1000 (400 RI)	1 mile *(1.5K)* easy 5 miles *(8K)* at MP 1 mile *(1.5K)* easy	20 miles at MP + 30 ***32K at MP + 19***
5	3 × 1600 (400 RI)	10 miles *(16K)* at MP	15 miles at MP + 15 ***24K at MP + 9***

WEEK	KEY RUN #1 (TRACK REPEATS)	KEY RUN #2 (TEMPO RUN)	KEY RUN #3 (LONG RUN)
4	10 × 400 (400 RI)	10 min warmup 8 miles *(13K)* at MP 10 min cooldown	20 miles at MP + 15 *32K at MP + 9*
3	8 × 800 (90 sec RI)	1 mile *(1.5K)* easy 5 miles *(8K)* at MT 1 mile *(1.5K)* easy	13 miles at MP *21K at MP*
2	5 × 1000 (400 RI)	2 miles *(3K)* easy 3 miles *(5K)* at ST 1 mile *(1.5K)* easy	10 miles at MP *16K at MP*
1	6 × 400 (400 RI)	10 min warmup 3 miles *(5K)* at MP 10 minute cooldown	Marathon 26.2 miles *(42.2K)*

Table 5.6

Key Run #1 (Track Repeats) Target Times
(improves economy, running speed, and VO_2max)

5K TIME	400M	600M	800M	1000M	1200M	1600M	2000M
0:16:00	0:01:07	0:01:43	0:02:18	0:02:55	0:03:34	0:04:53	0:06:11
0:16:10	0:01:08	0:01:44	0:02:20	0:02:57	0:03:36	0:04:56	0:06:15
0:16:20	0:01:09	0:01:45	0:02:22	0:02:59	0:03:39	0:04:59	0:06:19
0:16:30	0:01:10	0:01:46	0:02:23	0:03:01	0:03:41	0:05:03	0:06:23
0:16:40	0:01:10	0:01:48	0:02:25	0:03:03	0:03:43	0:05:06	0:06:27
0:16:50	0:01:11	0:01:49	0:02:27	0:03:05	0:03:46	0:05:09	0:06:31
0:17:00	0:01:12	0:01:50	0:02:28	0:03:07	0:03:48	0:05:12	0:06:35
0:17:10	0:01:13	0:01:51	0:02:30	0:03:09	0:03:51	0:05:16	0:06:39
0:17:20	0:01:14	0:01:53	0:02:31	0:03:11	0:03:53	0:05:19	0:06:43
0:17:30	0:01:14	0:01:54	0:02:33	0:03:13	0:03:55	0:05:22	0:06:47
0:17:40	0:01:15	0:01:55	0:02:35	0:03:15	0:03:58	0:05:25	0:06:51
0:17:50	0:01:16	0:01:56	0:02:36	0:03:17	0:04:00	0:05:28	0:06:55
0:18:00	0:01:17	0:01:57	0:02:38	0:03:19	0:04:03	0:05:32	0:07:00
0:18:10	0:01:18	0:01:59	0:02:39	0:03:21	0:04:05	0:05:35	0:07:04
0:18:20	0:01:19	0:02:00	0:02:41	0:03:23	0:04:08	0:05:38	0:07:08
0:18:30	0:01:19	0:02:01	0:02:43	0:03:25	0:04:10	0:05:41	0:07:12
0:18:40	0:01:20	0:02:02	0:02:44	0:03:27	0:04:12	0:05:44	0:07:16
0:18:50	0:01:21	0:02:03	0:02:46	0:03:29	0:04:15	0:05:48	0:07:20
0:19:00	0:01:22	0:02:05	0:02:47	0:03:31	0:04:17	0:05:51	0:07:24
0:19:10	0:01:23	0:02:06	0:02:49	0:03:33	0:04:20	0:05:54	0:07:28
0:19:20	0:01:23	0:02:07	0:02:51	0:03:35	0:04:22	0:05:57	0:07:32
0:19:30	0:01:24	0:02:08	0:02:52	0:03:37	0:04:24	0:06:01	0:07:36
0:19:40	0:01:25	0:02:09	0:02:54	0:03:39	0:04:27	0:06:04	0:07:40
0:19:50	0:01:26	0:02:11	0:02:56	0:03:41	0:04:29	0:06:07	0:07:44
0:20:00	0:01:27	0:02:12	0:02:57	0:03:43	0:04:32	0:06:10	0:07:48
0:20:10	0:01:27	0:02:13	0:02:59	0:03:45	0:04:34	0:06:13	0:07:52
0:20:20	0:01:28	0:02:14	0:03:00	0:03:47	0:04:36	0:06:17	0:07:56
0:20:30	0:01:29	0:02:15	0:03:02	0:03:49	0:04:39	0:06:20	0:08:00
0:20:40	0:01:30	0:02:17	0:03:04	0:03:51	0:04:41	0:06:23	0:08:04

5K TIME	400M	600M	800M	1000M	1200M	1600M	2000M
0:20:50	0:01:31	0:02:18	0:03:05	0:03:53	0:04:44	0:06:26	0:08:08
0:21:00	0:01:31	0:02:19	0:03:07	0:03:55	0:04:46	0:06:30	0:08:12
0:21:10	0:01:32	0:02:20	0:03:08	0:03:57	0:04:49	0:06:33	0:08:16
0:21:20	0:01:33	0:02:21	0:03:10	0:03:59	0:04:51	0:06:36	0:08:20
0:21:30	0:01:34	0:02:23	0:03:12	0:04:01	0:04:53	0:06:39	0:08:24
0:21:40	0:01:35	0:02:24	0:03:13	0:04:04	0:04:56	0:06:42	0:08:28
0:21:50	0:01:35	0:02:25	0:03:15	0:04:06	0:04:58	0:06:46	0:08:32
0:22:00	0:01:36	0:02:26	0:03:16	0:04:08	0:05:01	0:06:49	0:08:36
0:22:10	0:01:37	0:02:28	0:03:18	0:04:10	0:05:03	0:06:52	0:08:40
0:22:20	0:01:38	0:02:29	0:03:20	0:04:12	0:05:05	0:06:55	0:08:44
0:22:30	0:01:39	0:02:30	0:03:21	0:04:14	0:05:08	0:06:59	0:08:48
0:22:40	0:01:39	0:02:31	0:03:23	0:04:16	0:05:10	0:07:02	0:08:52
0:22:50	0:01:40	0:02:32	0:03:24	0:04:18	0:05:13	0:07:05	0:08:56
0:23:00	0:01:41	0:02:34	0:03:26	0:04:20	0:05:15	0:07:08	0:09:00
0:23:10	0:01:42	0:02:35	0:03:28	0:04:22	0:05:18	0:07:11	0:09:04
0:23:20	0:01:43	0:02:36	0:03:29	0:04:24	0:05:20	0:07:15	0:09:08
0:23:30	0:01:43	0:02:37	0:03:31	0:04:26	0:05:22	0:07:18	0:09:12
0:23:40	0:01:44	0:02:38	0:03:33	0:04:28	0:05:25	0:07:21	0:09:16
0:23:50	0:01:45	0:02:40	0:03:34	0:04:30	0:05:27	0:07:24	0:09:20
0:24:00	0:01:46	0:02:41	0:03:36	0:04:32	0:05:30	0:07:27	0:09:24
0:24:10	0:01:47	0:02:42	0:03:37	0:04:34	0:05:32	0:07:31	0:09:28
0:24:20	0:01:47	0:02:43	0:03:39	0:04:36	0:05:34	0:07:34	0:09:32
0:24:30	0:01:48	0:02:44	0:03:41	0:04:38	0:05:37	0:07:37	0:09:36
0:24:40	0:01:49	0:02:46	0:03:42	0:04:40	0:05:39	0:07:40	0:09:40
0:24:50	0:01:50	0:02:47	0:03:44	0:04:42	0:05:42	0:07:44	0:09:44
0:25:00	0:01:51	0:02:48	0:03:45	0:04:44	0:05:44	0:07:47	0:09:48
0:25:10	0:01:51	0:02:49	0:03:47	0:04:46	0:05:46	0:07:50	0:09:52
0:25:20	0:01:52	0:02:50	0:03:49	0:04:48	0:05:49	0:07:53	0:09:57
0:25:30	0:01:53	0:02:52	0:03:50	0:04:50	0:05:51	0:07:56	0:10:01

5K TIME	400M	600M	800M	1000M	1200M	1600M	2000M
0:25:40	0:01:54	0:02:53	0:03:52	0:04:52	0:05:54	0:08:00	0:10:05
0:25:50	0:01:55	0:02:54	0:03:53	0:04:54	0:05:56	0:08:03	0:10:09
0:26:00	0:01:56	0:02:55	0:03:55	0:04:56	0:05:59	0:08:06	0:10:13
0:26:10	0:01:56	0:02:56	0:03:57	0:04:58	0:06:01	0:08:09	0:10:17
0:26:20	0:01:57	0:02:58	0:03:58	0:05:00	0:06:03	0:08:13	0:10:21
0:26:30	0:01:58	0:02:59	0:04:00	0:05:02	0:06:06	0:08:16	0:10:25
0:26:40	0:01:59	0:03:00	0:04:01	0:05:04	0:06:08	0:08:19	0:10:29
0:26:50	0:02:00	0:03:01	0:04:03	0:05:06	0:06:11	0:08:22	0:10:33
0:27:00	0:02:00	0:03:03	0:04:05	0:05:08	0:06:13	0:08:25	0:10:37
0:27:10	0:02:01	0:03:04	0:04:06	0:05:10	0:06:15	0:08:29	0:10:41
0:27:20	0:02:02	0:03:05	0:04:08	0:05:12	0:06:18	0:08:32	0:10:45
0:27:30	0:02:03	0:03:06	0:04:10	0:05:14	0:06:20	0:08:35	0:10:49
0:27:40	0:02:04	0:03:07	0:04:11	0:05:16	0:06:23	0:08:38	0:10:53
0:27:50	0:02:04	0:03:09	0:04:13	0:05:18	0:06:25	0:08:41	0:10:57
0:28:00	0:02:05	0:03:10	0:04:14	0:05:20	0:06:28	0:08:45	0:11:01
0:28:10	0:02:06	0:03:11	0:04:16	0:05:22	0:06:30	0:08:48	0:11:05
0:28:20	0:02:07	0:03:12	0:04:18	0:05:24	0:06:32	0:08:51	0:11:09
0:28:30	0:02:08	0:03:13	0:04:19	0:05:26	0:06:35	0:08:54	0:11:13
0:28:40	0:02:08	0:03:15	0:04:21	0:05:28	0:06:37	0:08:58	0:11:17
0:28:50	0:02:09	0:03:16	0:04:22	0:05:30	0:06:40	0:09:01	0:11:21
0:29:00	0:02:10	0:03:17	0:04:24	0:05:32	0:06:42	0:09:04	0:11:25
0:29:10	0:02:11	0:03:18	0:04:26	0:05:34	0:06:44	0:09:07	0:11:29
0:29:20	0:02:12	0:03:19	0:04:27	0:05:36	0:06:47	0:09:10	0:11:33
0:29:30	0:02:12	0:03:21	0:04:29	0:05:38	0:06:49	0:09:14	0:11:37
0:29:40	0:02:13	0:03:22	0:04:30	0:05:40	0:06:52	0:09:17	0:11:41
0:29:50	0:02:14	0:03:23	0:04:32	0:05:42	0:06:54	0:09:20	0:11:45
0:30:00	0:02:15	0:03:24	0:04:34	0:05:44	0:06:57	0:09:23	0:11:49
0:30:10	0:02:16	0:03:25	0:04:35	0:05:46	0:06:59	0:09:27	0:11:53
0:30:20	0:02:16	0:03:27	0:04:37	0:05:48	0:07:01	0:09:30	0:11:57
0:30:30	0:02:17	0:03:28	0:04:38	0:05:50	0:07:04	0:09:33	0:12:01
0:30:40	0:02:18	0:03:29	0:04:40	0:05:52	0:07:06	0:09:36	0:12:05
0:30:50	0:02:19	0:03:30	0:04:42	0:05:54	0:07:09	0:09:39	0:12:09

5K TIME	400M	600M	800M	1000M	1200M	1600M	2000M
0:31:00	0:02:20	0:03:31	0:04:43	0:05:56	0:07:11	0:09:43	0:12:13
0:31:10	0:02:20	0:03:33	0:04:45	0:05:58	0:07:13	0:09:46	0:12:17
0:31:20	0:02:21	0:03:34	0:04:47	0:06:00	0:07:16	0:09:49	0:12:21
0:31:30	0:02:22	0:03:35	0:04:48	0:06:02	0:07:18	0:09:52	0:12:25
0:31:40	0:02:23	0:03:36	0:04:50	0:06:04	0:07:21	0:09:56	0:12:29
0:31:50	0:02:24	0:03:38	0:04:51	0:06:06	0:07:23	0:09:59	0:12:33
0:32:00	0:02:24	0:03:39	0:04:53	0:06:08	0:07:25	0:10:02	0:12:37
0:32:10	0:02:25	0:03:40	0:04:55	0:06:10	0:07:28	0:10:05	0:12:41
0:32:20	0:02:26	0:03:41	0:04:56	0:06:12	0:07:30	0:10:08	0:12:45
0:32:30	0:02:27	0:03:42	0:04:58	0:06:14	0:07:33	0:10:12	0:12:50
0:32:40	0:02:28	0:03:44	0:04:59	0:06:16	0:07:35	0:10:15	0:12:54
0:32:50	0:02:29	0:03:45	0:05:01	0:06:18	0:07:38	0:10:18	0:12:58
0:33:00	0:02:29	0:03:46	0:05:03	0:06:20	0:07:40	0:10:21	0:13:02
0:33:10	0:02:30	0:03:47	0:05:04	0:06:22	0:07:42	0:10:24	0:13:06
0:33:20	0:02:31	0:03:48	0:05:06	0:06:24	0:07:45	0:10:28	0:13:10
0:33:30	0:02:32	0:03:50	0:05:07	0:06:26	0:07:47	0:10:31	0:13:14
0:33:40	0:02:33	0:03:51	0:05:09	0:06:28	0:07:50	0:10:34	0:13:18
0:33:50	0:02:33	0:03:52	0:05:11	0:06:30	0:07:52	0:10:37	0:13:22
0:34:00	0:02:34	0:03:53	0:05:12	0:06:32	0:07:54	0:10:41	0:13:26
0:34:10	0:02:35	0:03:54	0:05:14	0:06:34	0:07:57	0:10:44	0:13:30
0:34:20	0:02:36	0:03:56	0:05:16	0:06:36	0:07:59	0:10:47	0:13:34
0:34:30	0:02:37	0:03:57	0:05:17	0:06:38	0:08:02	0:10:50	0:13:38
0:34:40	0:02:37	0:03:58	0:05:19	0:06:40	0:08:04	0:10:53	0:13:42
0:34:50	0:02:38	0:03:59	0:05:20	0:06:42	0:08:07	0:10:57	0:13:46
0:35:00	0:02:39	0:04:00	0:05:22	0:06:44	0:08:09	0:11:00	0:13:50
0:35:10	0:02:40	0:04:02	0:05:24	0:06:46	0:08:11	0:11:03	0:13:54
0:35:20	0:02:41	0:04:03	0:05:25	0:06:48	0:08:14	0:11:06	0:13:58
0:35:30	0:02:41	0:04:04	0:05:27	0:06:50	0:08:16	0:11:10	0:14:02
0:35:40	0:02:42	0:04:05	0:05:28	0:06:52	0:08:19	0:11:13	0:14:06
0:35:50	0:02:43	0:04:06	0:05:30	0:06:54	0:08:21	0:11:16	0:14:10
0:36:00	0:02:44	0:04:08	0:05:32	0:06:57	0:08:23	0:11:19	0:14:14
0:36:10	0:02:45	0:04:09	0:05:33	0:06:59	0:08:26	0:11:22	0:14:18

5K TIME	400M	600M	800M	1000M	1200M	1600M	2000M
0:36:20	0:02:45	0:04:10	0:05:35	0:07:01	0:08:28	0:11:26	0:14:22
0:36:30	0:02:46	0:04:11	0:05:36	0:07:03	0:08:31	0:11:29	0:14:26
0:36:40	0:02:47	0:04:13	0:05:38	0:07:05	0:08:33	0:11:32	0:14:30
0:36:50	0:02:48	0:04:14	0:05:40	0:07:07	0:08:35	0:11:35	0:14:34
0:37:00	0:02:49	0:04:15	0:05:41	0:07:09	0:08:38	0:11:39	0:14:38
0:37:10	0:02:49	0:04:16	0:05:43	0:07:11	0:08:40	0:11:42	0:14:42
0:37:20	0:02:50	0:04:17	0:05:44	0:07:13	0:08:43	0:11:45	0:14:46
0:37:30	0:02:51	0:04:19	0:05:46	0:07:15	0:08:45	0:11:48	0:14:50
0:37:40	0:02:52	0:04:20	0:05:48	0:07:17	0:08:48	0:11:51	0:14:54
0:37:50	0:02:53	0:04:21	0:05:49	0:07:19	0:08:50	0:11:55	0:14:58
0:38:00	0:02:53	0:04:22	0:05:51	0:07:21	0:08:52	0:11:58	0:15:02
0:38:10	0:02:54	0:04:23	0:05:53	0:07:23	0:08:55	0:12:01	0:15:06
0:38:20	0:02:55	0:04:25	0:05:54	0:07:25	0:08:57	0:12:04	0:15:10
0:38:30	0:02:56	0:04:26	0:05:56	0:07:27	0:09:00	0:12:07	0:15:14
0:38:40	0:02:57	0:04:27	0:05:57	0:07:29	0:09:02	0:12:11	0:15:18
0:38:50	0:02:57	0:04:28	0:05:59	0:07:31	0:09:04	0:12:14	0:15:22
0:39:00	0:02:58	0:04:29	0:06:01	0:07:33	0:09:07	0:12:17	0:15:26
0:39:10	0:02:59	0:04:31	0:06:02	0:07:35	0:09:09	0:12:20	0:15:30
0:39:20	0:03:00	0:04:32	0:06:04	0:07:37	0:09:12	0:12:24	0:15:34
0:39:30	0:03:01	0:04:33	0:06:05	0:07:39	0:09:14	0:12:27	0:15:38
0:39:40	0:03:02	0:04:34	0:06:07	0:07:41	0:09:17	0:12:30	0:15:43
0:39:50	0:03:02	0:04:35	0:06:09	0:07:43	0:09:19	0:12:33	0:15:47
0:40:00	0:03:03	0:04:37	0:06:10	0:07:45	0:09:21	0:12:36	0:15:51

Table 5.7

Key Run #2 (Tempo Run) Paces
(improves lactate tolerance)

	(PER MILE)			(PER KILOMETER)		
5K TIME	**SHORT TEMPO**	**MID TEMPO**	**LONG TEMPO**	**SHORT TEMPO**	**MID TEMPO**	**LONG TEMPO**
0:16:00	0:05:26	0:05:41	0:05:56	0:03:22	0:03:32	0:03:41
0:16:10	0:05:29	0:05:44	0:05:59	0:03:24	0:03:34	0:03:43
0:16:20	0:05:32	0:05:47	0:06:02	0:03:26	0:03:36	0:03:45
0:16:30	0:05:36	0:05:51	0:06:06	0:03:28	0:03:38	0:03:47
0:16:40	0:05:39	0:05:54	0:06:09	0:03:30	0:03:40	0:03:49
0:16:50	0:05:42	0:05:57	0:06:12	0:03:32	0:03:42	0:03:51
0:17:00	0:05:45	0:06:00	0:06:15	0:03:34	0:03:44	0:03:53
0:17:10	0:05:49	0:06:04	0:06:19	0:03:36	0:03:46	0:03:55
0:17:20	0:05:52	0:06:07	0:06:22	0:03:38	0:03:48	0:03:57
0:17:30	0:05:55	0:06:10	0:06:25	0:03:40	0:03:50	0:03:59
0:17:40	0:05:58	0:06:13	0:06:28	0:03:42	0:03:52	0:04:01
0:17:50	0:06:01	0:06:16	0:06:31	0:03:44	0:03:54	0:04:03
0:18:00	0:06:05	0:06:20	0:06:35	0:03:46	0:03:56	0:04:05
0:18:10	0:06:08	0:06:23	0:06:38	0:03:48	0:03:58	0:04:07
0:18:20	0:06:11	0:06:26	0:06:41	0:03:50	0:04:00	0:04:09
0:18:30	0:06:14	0:06:29	0:06:44	0:03:52	0:04:02	0:04:11
0:18:40	0:06:17	0:06:32	0:06:47	0:03:54	0:04:04	0:04:13
0:18:50	0:06:21	0:06:36	0:06:51	0:03:56	0:04:06	0:04:15
0:19:00	0:06:24	0:06:39	0:06:54	0:03:58	0:04:08	0:04:17
0:19:10	0:06:27	0:06:42	0:06:57	0:04:00	0:04:10	0:04:19
0:19:20	0:06:30	0:06:45	0:07:00	0:04:02	0:04:12	0:04:21
0:19:30	0:06:34	0:06:49	0:07:04	0:04:04	0:04:14	0:04:23
0:19:40	0:06:37	0:06:52	0:07:07	0:04:06	0:04:16	0:04:25
0:19:50	0:06:40	0:06:55	0:07:10	0:04:08	0:04:18	0:04:27
0:20:00	0:06:43	0:06:58	0:07:13	0:04:10	0:04:20	0:04:29
0:20:10	0:06:46	0:07:01	0:07:16	0:04:12	0:04:22	0:04:31
0:20:20	0:06:50	0:07:05	0:07:20	0:04:14	0:04:24	0:04:33
0:20:30	0:06:53	0:07:08	0:07:23	0:04:16	0:04:26	0:04:35

	(PER MILE)			(PER KILOMETER)		
5k TIME	**SHORT TEMPO**	**MID TEMPO**	**LONG TEMPO**	**SHORT TEMPO**	**MID TEMPO**	**LONG TEMPO**
0:20:40	0:06:56	0:07:11	0:07:26	0:04:18	0:04:28	0:04:37
0:20:50	0:06:59	0:07:14	0:07:29	0:04:20	0:04:30	0:04:39
0:21:00	0:07:03	0:07:18	0:07:33	0:04:22	0:04:32	0:04:41
0:21:10	0:07:06	0:07:21	0:07:36	0:04:24	0:04:34	0:04:43
0:21:20	0:07:09	0:07:24	0:07:39	0:04:26	0:04:36	0:04:45
0:21:30	0:07:12	0:07:27	0:07:42	0:04:28	0:04:38	0:04:47
0:21:40	0:07:15	0:07:30	0:07:45	0:04:30	0:04:40	0:04:49
0:21:50	0:07:19	0:07:34	0:07:49	0:04:32	0:04:42	0:04:51
0:22:00	0:07:22	0:07:37	0:07:52	0:04:34	0:04:44	0:04:53
0:22:10	0:07:25	0:07:40	0:07:55	0:04:36	0:04:46	0:04:55
0:22:20	0:07:28	0:07:43	0:07:58	0:04:38	0:04:48	0:04:57
0:22:30	0:07:32	0:07:47	0:08:02	0:04:40	0:04:50	0:04:59
0:22:40	0:07:35	0:07:50	0:08:05	0:04:42	0:04:52	0:05:01
0:22:50	0:07:38	0:07:53	0:08:08	0:04:44	0:04:54	0:05:03
0:23:00	0:07:41	0:07:56	0:08:11	0:04:46	0:04:56	0:05:05
0:23:10	0:07:44	0:07:59	0:08:14	0:04:48	0:04:58	0:05:07
0:23:20	0:07:48	0:08:03	0:08:18	0:04:50	0:05:00	0:05:09
0:23:30	0:07:51	0:08:06	0:08:21	0:04:52	0:05:02	0:05:11
0:23:40	0:07:54	0:08:09	0:08:24	0:04:54	0:05:04	0:05:13
0:23:50	0:07:57	0:08:12	0:08:27	0:04:56	0:05:06	0:05:15
0:24:00	0:08:00	0:08:15	0:08:30	0:04:58	0:05:08	0:05:17
0:24:10	0:08:04	0:08:19	0:08:34	0:05:00	0:05:10	0:05:19
0:24:20	0:08:07	0:08:22	0:08:37	0:05:02	0:05:12	0:05:21
0:24:30	0:08:10	0:08:25	0:08:40	0:05:04	0:05:14	0:05:23
0:24:40	0:08:13	0:08:28	0:08:43	0:05:06	0:05:16	0:05:25
0:24:50	0:08:17	0:08:32	0:08:47	0:05:08	0:05:18	0:05:27
0:25:00	0:08:20	0:08:35	0:08:50	0:05:10	0:05:20	0:05:29
0:25:10	0:08:23	0:08:38	0:08:53	0:05:12	0:05:22	0:05:31
0:25:20	0:08:26	0:08:41	0:08:56	0:05:14	0:05:24	0:05:33
0:25:30	0:08:29	0:08:44	0:08:59	0:05:16	0:05:26	0:05:35
0:25:40	0:08:33	0:08:48	0:09:03	0:05:18	0:05:28	0:05:37

5k TIME	(PER MILE)			(PER KILOMETER)		
	SHORT TEMPO	MID TEMPO	LONG TEMPO	SHORT TEMPO	MID TEMPO	LONG TEMPO
0:25:50	0:08:36	0:08:51	0:09:06	0:05:20	0:05:30	0:05:39
0:26:00	0:08:39	0:08:54	0:09:09	0:05:22	0:05:32	0:05:41
0:26:10	0:08:42	0:08:57	0:09:12	0:05:24	0:05:34	0:05:43
0:26:20	0:08:46	0:09:01	0:09:16	0:05:26	0:05:36	0:05:45
0:26:30	0:08:49	0:09:04	0:09:19	0:05:28	0:05:38	0:05:47
0:26:40	0:08:52	0:09:07	0:09:22	0:05:30	0:05:40	0:05:49
0:26:50	0:08:55	0:09:10	0:09:25	0:05:32	0:05:42	0:05:51
0:27:00	0:08:58	0:09:13	0:09:28	0:05:34	0:05:44	0:05:53
0:27:10	0:09:02	0:09:17	0:09:32	0:05:36	0:05:46	0:05:55
0:27:20	0:09:05	0:09:20	0:09:35	0:05:38	0:05:48	0:05:57
0:27:30	0:09:08	0:09:23	0:09:38	0:05:40	0:05:50	0:05:59
0:27:40	0:09:11	0:09:26	0:09:41	0:05:42	0:05:52	0:06:01
0:27:50	0:09:14	0:09:29	0:09:44	0:05:44	0:05:54	0:06:03
0:28:00	0:09:18	0:09:33	0:09:48	0:05:46	0:05:56	0:06:05
0:28:10	0:09:21	0:09:36	0:09:51	0:05:48	0:05:58	0:06:07
0:28:20	0:09:24	0:09:39	0:09:54	0:05:50	0:06:00	0:06:09
0:28:30	0:09:27	0:09:42	0:09:57	0:05:52	0:06:02	0:06:11
0:28:40	0:09:31	0:09:46	0:10:01	0:05:54	0:06:04	0:06:13
0:28:50	0:09:34	0:09:49	0:10:04	0:05:56	0:06:06	0:06:15
0:29:00	0:09:37	0:09:52	0:10:07	0:05:58	0:06:08	0:06:17
0:29:10	0:09:40	0:09:55	0:10:10	0:06:00	0:06:10	0:06:19
0:29:20	0:09:43	0:09:58	0:10:13	0:06:02	0:06:12	0:06:21
0:29:30	0:09:47	0:10:02	0:10:17	0:06:04	0:06:14	0:06:23
0:29:40	0:09:50	0:10:05	0:10:20	0:06:06	0:06:16	0:06:25
0:29:50	0:09:53	0:10:08	0:10:23	0:06:08	0:06:18	0:06:27
0:30:00	0:09:56	0:10:11	0:10:26	0:06:10	0:06:20	0:06:29
0:30:10	0:10:00	0:10:15	0:10:30	0:06:12	0:06:22	0:06:31
0:30:20	0:10:03	0:10:18	0:10:33	0:06:14	0:06:24	0:06:33
0:30:30	0:10:06	0:10:21	0:10:36	0:06:16	0:06:26	0:06:35
0:30:40	0:10:09	0:10:24	0:10:39	0:06:18	0:06:28	0:06:37
0:30:50	0:10:12	0:10:27	0:10:42	0:06:20	0:06:30	0:06:39

	(PER MILE)			(PER KILOMETER)		
5K TIME	**SHORT TEMPO**	**MID TEMPO**	**LONG TEMPO**	**SHORT TEMPO**	**MID TEMPO**	**LONG TEMPO**
0:31:00	0:10:16	0:10:31	0:10:46	0:06:22	0:06:32	0:06:41
0:31:10	0:10:19	0:10:34	0:10:49	0:06:24	0:06:34	0:06:43
0:31:20	0:10:22	0:10:37	0:10:52	0:06:26	0:06:36	0:06:45
0:31:30	0:10:25	0:10:40	0:10:55	0:06:28	0:06:38	0:06:47
0:31:40	0:10:29	0:10:44	0:10:59	0:06:30	0:06:40	0:06:49
0:31:50	0:10:32	0:10:47	0:11:02	0:06:32	0:06:42	0:06:51
0:32:00	0:10:35	0:10:50	0:11:05	0:06:34	0:06:44	0:06:53
0:32:10	0:10:38	0:10:53	0:11:08	0:06:36	0:06:46	0:06:55
0:32:20	0:10:41	0:10:56	0:11:11	0:06:38	0:06:48	0:06:57
0:32:30	0:10:45	0:11:00	0:11:15	0:06:40	0:06:50	0:06:59
0:32:40	0:10:48	0:11:03	0:11:18	0:06:42	0:06:52	0:07:01
0:32:50	0:10:51	0:11:06	0:11:21	0:06:44	0:06:54	0:07:03
0:33:00	0:10:54	0:11:09	0:11:24	0:06:46	0:06:56	0:07:05
0:33:10	0:10:57	0:11:12	0:11:27	0:06:48	0:06:58	0:07:07
0:33:20	0:11:01	0:11:16	0:11:31	0:06:50	0:07:00	0:07:09
0:33:30	0:11:04	0:11:19	0:11:34	0:06:52	0:07:02	0:07:11
0:33:40	0:11:07	0:11:22	0:11:37	0:06:54	0:07:04	0:07:13
0:33:50	0:11:10	0:11:25	0:11:40	0:06:56	0:07:06	0:07:15
0:34:00	0:11:14	0:11:29	0:11:44	0:06:58	0:07:08	0:07:17
0:34:10	0:11:17	0:11:32	0:11:47	0:07:00	0:07:10	0:07:19
0:34:20	0:11:20	0:11:35	0:11:50	0:07:02	0:07:12	0:07:21
0:34:30	0:11:23	0:11:38	0:11:53	0:07:04	0:07:14	0:07:23
0:34:40	0:11:26	0:11:41	0:11:56	0:07:06	0:07:16	0:07:25
0:34:50	0:11:30	0:11:45	0:12:00	0:07:08	0:07:18	0:07:27
0:35:00	0:11:33	0:11:48	0:12:03	0:07:10	0:07:20	0:07:29
0:35:10	0:11:36	0:11:51	0:12:06	0:07:12	0:07:22	0:07:31
0:35:20	0:11:39	0:11:54	0:12:09	0:07:14	0:07:24	0:07:33
0:35:30	0:11:43	0:11:58	0:12:13	0:07:16	0:07:26	0:07:35

	(PER MILE)			(PER KILOMETER)		
5K TIME	**SHORT TEMPO**	**MID TEMPO**	**LONG TEMPO**	**SHORT TEMPO**	**MID TEMPO**	**LONG TEMPO**
0:35:40	0:11:46	0:12:01	0:12:16	0:07:18	0:07:28	0:07:37
0:35:50	0:11:49	0:12:04	0:12:19	0:07:20	0:07:30	0:07:39
0:36:00	0:11:52	0:12:07	0:12:22	0:07:22	0:07:32	0:07:41
0:36:10	0:11:55	0:12:10	0:12:25	0:07:24	0:07:34	0:07:43
0:36:20	0:11:59	0:12:14	0:12:29	0:07:26	0:07:36	0:07:45
0:36:30	0:12:02	0:12:17	0:12:32	0:07:28	0:07:38	0:07:47
0:36:40	0:12:05	0:12:20	0:12:35	0:07:30	0:07:40	0:07:49
0:36:50	0:12:08	0:12:23	0:12:38	0:07:32	0:07:42	0:07:51
0:37:00	0:12:12	0:12:27	0:12:42	0:07:34	0:07:44	0:07:53
0:37:10	0:12:15	0:12:30	0:12:45	0:07:36	0:07:46	0:07:55
0:37:20	0:12:18	0:12:33	0:12:48	0:07:38	0:07:48	0:07:57
0:37:30	0:12:21	0:12:36	0:12:51	0:07:40	0:07:50	0:07:59
0:37:40	0:12:24	0:12:39	0:12:54	0:07:42	0:07:52	0:08:01
0:37:50	0:12:28	0:12:43	0:12:58	0:07:44	0:07:54	0:08:03
0:38:00	0:12:31	0:12:46	0:13:01	0:07:46	0:07:56	0:08:05
0:38:10	0:12:34	0:12:49	0:13:04	0:07:48	0:07:58	0:08:07
0:38:20	0:12:37	0:12:52	0:13:07	0:07:50	0:08:00	0:08:09
0:38:30	0:12:40	0:12:55	0:13:10	0:07:52	0:08:02	0:08:11
0:38:40	0:12:44	0:12:59	0:13:14	0:07:54	0:08:04	0:08:13
0:38:50	0:12:47	0:13:02	0:13:17	0:07:56	0:08:06	0:08:15
0:39:00	0:12:50	0:13:05	0:13:20	0:07:58	0:08:08	0:08:17
0:39:10	0:12:53	0:13:08	0:13:23	0:08:00	0:08:10	0:08:19
0:39:20	0:12:57	0:13:12	0:13:27	0:08:02	0:08:12	0:08:21
0:39:30	0:13:00	0:13:15	0:13:30	0:08:04	0:08:14	0:08:23
0:39:40	0:13:03	0:13:18	0:13:33	0:08:06	0:08:16	0:08:25
0:39:50	0:13:06	0:13:21	0:13:36	0:08:08	0:08:18	0:08:27
0:40:00	0:13:09	0:13:24	0:13:39	0:08:10	0:08:20	0:08:29

Table 5.8

Key Run #3 (Long Run) Paces
(improves skeletal and cardiac muscle adaptation)

5ᴋ TIME	(PER MILE)		(PER KILOMETER)	
	MP	HMP	MP	HMP
0:16:00	0:05:56	0:05:39	0:03:41	0:03:31
0:16:10	0:06:00	0:05:43	0:03:44	0:03:33
0:16:20	0:06:04	0:05:46	0:03:46	0:03:35
0:16:30	0:06:07	0:05:50	0:03:48	0:03:38
0:16:40	0:06:11	0:05:54	0:03:51	0:03:40
0:16:50	0:06:15	0:05:57	0:03:53	0:03:42
0:17:00	0:06:19	0:06:01	0:03:55	0:03:44
0:17:10	0:06:22	0:06:04	0:03:58	0:03:46
0:17:20	0:06:26	0:06:08	0:04:00	0:03:48
0:17:30	0:06:30	0:06:11	0:04:02	0:03:51
0:17:40	0:06:33	0:06:15	0:04:04	0:03:53
0:17:50	0:06:37	0:06:18	0:04:07	0:03:55
0:18:00	0:06:41	0:06:22	0:04:09	0:03:57
0:18:10	0:06:45	0:06:25	0:04:11	0:03:59
0:18:20	0:06:48	0:06:29	0:04:14	0:04:02
0:18:30	0:06:52	0:06:32	0:04:16	0:04:04
0:18:40	0:06:56	0:06:36	0:04:18	0:04:06
0:18:50	0:06:59	0:06:40	0:04:21	0:04:08
0:19:00	0:07:03	0:06:43	0:04:23	0:04:10
0:19:10	0:07:07	0:06:47	0:04:25	0:04:13
0:19:20	0:07:11	0:06:50	0:04:28	0:04:15
0:19:30	0:07:14	0:06:54	0:04:30	0:04:17
0:19:40	0:07:18	0:06:57	0:04:32	0:04:19
0:19:50	0:07:22	0:07:01	0:04:34	0:04:21
0:20:00	0:07:25	0:07:04	0:04:37	0:04:24
0:20:10	0:07:29	0:07:08	0:04:39	0:04:26
0:20:20	0:07:33	0:07:11	0:04:41	0:04:28
0:20:30	0:07:37	0:07:15	0:04:44	0:04:30

	(PER MILE)		(PER KILOMETER)	
5K TIME	**MP**	**HMP**	**MP**	**HMP**
0:20:40	0:07:40	0:07:18	0:04:46	0:04:32
0:20:50	0:07:44	0:07:22	0:04:48	0:04:35
0:21:00	0:07:48	0:07:25	0:04:51	0:04:37
0:21:10	0:07:51	0:07:29	0:04:53	0:04:39
0:21:20	0:07:55	0:07:33	0:04:55	0:04:41
0:21:30	0:07:59	0:07:36	0:04:58	0:04:43
0:21:40	0:08:02	0:07:40	0:05:00	0:04:46
0:21:50	0:08:06	0:07:43	0:05:02	0:04:48
0:22:00	0:08:10	0:07:47	0:05:04	0:04:50
0:22:10	0:08:14	0:07:50	0:05:07	0:04:52
0:22:20	0:08:17	0:07:54	0:05:09	0:04:54
0:22:30	0:08:21	0:07:57	0:05:11	0:04:57
0:22:40	0:08:23	0:08:01	0:05:14	0:04:59
0:22:50	0:08:28	0:08:04	0:05:16	0:05:01
0:23:00	0:08:32	0:08:08	0:05:18	0:05:03
0:23:10	0:08:36	0:08:11	0:05:21	0:05:05
0:23:20	0:08:40	0:08:15	0:05:23	0:05:08
0:23:30	0:08:43	0:08:19	0:05:25	0:05:10
0:23:40	0:08:47	0:08:22	0:05:27	0:05:12
0:23:50	0:08:51	0:08:26	0:05:30	0:05:14
0:24:00	0:08:54	0:08:29	0:05:32	0:05:16
0:24:10	0:08:58	0:08:33	0:05:34	0:05:19
0:24:20	0:09:02	0:08:36	0:05:37	0:05:21
0:24:30	0:09:06	0:08:40	0:05:39	0:05:23
0:24:40	0:09:09	0:08:43	0:05:41	0:05:25
0:24:50	0:09:13	0:08:47	0:05:44	0:05:27
0:25:00	0:09:17	0:08:50	0:05:46	0:05:30
0:25:10	0:09:20	0:08:54	0:05:48	0:05:32

	(PER MILE)		(PER KILOMETER)	
5K TIME	MP	HMP	MP	HMP
0:25:20	0:09:24	0:08:57	0:05:51	0:05:34
0:25:30	0:09:28	0:09:01	0:05:53	0:05:36
0:25:40	0:09:32	0:09:04	0:05:55	0:05:38
0:25:50	0:09:35	0:09:08	0:05:57	0:05:41
0:26:00	0:09:39	0:09:12	0:06:00	0:05:43
0:26:10	0:09:43	0:09:15	0:06:02	0:05:45
0:26:20	0:09:46	0:09:19	0:06:04	0:05:47
0:26:30	0:09:50	0:09:22	0:06:07	0:05:49
0:26:40	0:09:54	0:09:26	0:06:09	0:05:52
0:26:50	0:09:58	0:09:29	0:06:11	0:05:54
0:27:00	0:10:01	0:09:33	0:06:14	0:05:56
0:27:10	0:10:05	0:09:36	0:06:16	0:05:58
0:27:20	0:10:09	0:09:40	0:06:18	0:06:00
0:27:30	0:10:12	0:09:43	0:06:21	0:06:03
0:27:40	0:10:16	0:09:47	0:06:23	0:06:05
0:27:50	0:10:20	0:09:50	0:06:25	0:06:07
0:28:00	0:10:24	0:09:54	0:06:27	0:06:09
0:28:10	0:10:27	0:09:58	0:06:30	0:06:11
0:28:20	0:10:31	0:10:01	0:06:32	0:06:13
0:28:30	0:10:35	0:10:05	0:06:34	0:06:16
0:28:40	0:10:38	0:10:08	0:06:37	0:06:18
0:28:50	0:10:42	0:10:12	0:06:39	0:06:20
0:29:00	0:10:46	0:10:15	0:06:41	0:06:22
0:29:10	0:10:50	0:10:19	0:06:44	0:06:24
0:29:20	0:10:53	0:10:22	0:06:46	0:06:27
0:29:30	0:10:57	0:10:26	0:06:48	0:06:29
0:29:40	0:11:01	0:10:29	0:06:51	0:06:31
0:29:50	0:11:04	0:10:33	0:06:53	0:06:33
0:30:00	0:11:08	0:10:36	0:06:55	0:06:35
0:30:10	0:11:12	0:10:40	0:06:57	0:06:38
0:30:20	0:11:15	0:10:43	0:07:00	0:06:40
0:30:30	0:11:19	0:10:47	0:07:02	0:06:42

	(PER MILE)		(PER KILOMETER)	
5K TIME	MP	HMP	MP	HMP
0:30:40	0:11:23	0:10:51	0:07:04	0:06:44
0:30:50	0:11:27	0:10:54	0:07:07	0:06:46
0:31:00	0:11:30	0:10:58	0:07:09	0:06:49
0:31:10	0:11:34	0:11:01	0:07:11	0:06:51
0:31:20	0:11:38	0:11:05	0:07:14	0:06:53
0:31:30	0:11:41	0:11:08	0:07:16	0:06:55
0:31:40	0:11:45	0:11:12	0:07:18	0:06:57
0:31:50	0:11:49	0:11:15	0:07:20	0:07:00
0:32:00	0:11:53	0:11:19	0:07:23	0:07:02
0:32:10	0:11:56	0:11:22	0:07:25	0:07:04
0:32:20	0:12:00	0:11:26	0:07:27	0:07:06
0:32:30	0:12:04	0:11:29	0:07:30	0:07:08
0:32:40	0:12:07	0:11:33	0:07:32	0:07:11
0:32:50	0:12:11	0:11:37	0:07:34	0:07:13
0:33:00	0:12:15	0:11:40	0:07:37	0:07:15
0:33:10	0:12:19	0:11:44	0:07:39	0:07:17
0:33:20	0:12:22	0:11:47	0:07:41	0:07:19
0:33:30	0:12:26	0:11:51	0:07:44	0:07:22
0:33:40	0:12:30	0:11:54	0:07:46	0:07:24
0:33:50	0:12:33	0:11:58	0:07:48	0:07:26
0:34:00	0:12:37	0:12:01	0:07:50	0:07:28
0:34:10	0:12:41	0:12:05	0:07:53	0:07:30
0:34:20	0:12:45	0:12:08	0:07:55	0:07:33
0:34:30	0:12:48	0:12:12	0:07:57	0:07:35
0:34:40	0:12:52	0:12:15	0:08:00	0:07:37
0:34:50	0:12:56	0:12:19	0:08:02	0:07:39
0:35:00	0:12:59	0:12:22	0:08:04	0:07:41
0:35:10	0:13:03	0:12:26	0:08:07	0:07:44
0:35:20	0:13:07	0:12:30	0:08:09	0:07:46
0:35:30	0:13:11	0:12:33	0:08:11	0:07:48
0:35:40	0:13:14	0:12:37	0:08:14	0:07:50
0:35:50	0:13:18	0:12:40	0:08:16	0:07:52

	(PER MILE)		(PER KILOMETER)	
5k TIME	**MP**	**HMP**	**MP**	**HMP**
0:36:00	0:13:22	0:12:44	0:08:18	0:07:55
0:36:10	0:13:25	0:12:47	0:08:20	0:07:57
0:36:20	0:13:29	0:12:51	0:08:23	0:07:59
0:36:30	0:13:33	0:12:54	0:08:25	0:08:01
0:36:40	0:13:37	0:12:58	0:08:27	0:08:03
0:36:50	0:13:40	0:13:01	0:08:30	0:08:06
0:37:00	0:13:44	0:13:05	0:08:32	0:08:08
0:37:10	0:13:48	0:13:08	0:08:34	0:08:10
0:37:20	0:13:51	0:13:12	0:08:37	0:08:12
0:37:30	0:13:55	0:13:16	0:08:39	0:08:14
0:37:40	0:13:59	0:13:19	0:08:41	0:08:17
0:37:50	0:14:03	0:13:23	0:08:44	0:08:19
0:38:00	0:14:06	0:13:26	0:08:46	0:08:21
0:38:10	0:14:10	0:13:30	0:08:48	0:08:23
0:38:20	0:14:14	0:13:33	0:08:50	0:08:25
0:38:30	0:14:17	0:13:37	0:08:53	0:08:28
0:38:40	0:14:21	0:13:40	0:08:55	0:08:30
0:38:50	0:14:25	0:13:44	0:08:57	0:08:32
0:39:00	0:14:28	0:13:47	0:09:00	0:08:34
0:39:10	0:14:32	0:13:51	0:09:02	0:08:36
0:39:20	0:14:36	0:13:54	0:09:04	0:08:38
0:39:30	0:14:40	0:13:58	0:09:07	0:08:41
0:39:40	0:14:43	0:14:01	0:09:09	0:08:43
0:39:50	0:14:47	0:14:05	0:09:11	0:08:45
0:40:00	0:14:51	0:14:09	0:09:13	0:08:47

TRAINING WITH PURPOSE: Q AND A

Q. When can I start the FIRST training program?

A. We recommend a base training of 15 miles per week for 3 months prior to beginning any of the FIRST programs; the base training for the marathon training program should be closer to 25 miles per week. In addition to the requisite weekly miles, runners must be capable of long runs of 5 miles for the 5K program, 6 miles for the 10K, 8 miles for the half-marathon and novice marathon, and 15 miles for the marathon training program. If you are a beginning runner, see Chapter 3.

Q. I have never done this type of training. How do I get started?

A. During the base training, gradually become familiar with the track repeats and tempo runs. By introducing just one of the faster-paced workouts at a time, you can avoid too great a training overload at one time. During the base training, these faster-paced workouts do not have to be run at a pace as fast as prescribed by FIRST for the training program. Use the 3-month base training to gradually work up to your FIRST training paces.

Q. Can I use my goal race times to determine my training paces?

A. It is important that training paces be determined from actual race time performances, which represent the runner's current fitness level. It needs to be emphasized that you should run the paces **based on your current fitness level** and not your goal race times. To do otherwise may increase your risk of a running-related injury.

We have coached runners who insist on trying to run training paces consistent with their goal race times rather than those determined from recent race performances, which reflect your fitness level. When runners try to maintain their ambitious training paces over several workouts, they run into problems. They may be able to do it for Key Run #1 and, perhaps, even Key Run #2, but then fall apart in Key Run #3. In Chapter 10, we address running-related injuries due to overly ambitious training paces.

Q. How important is it to stick to the prescribed paces?

A. Very important. Running more slowly will not provide the stimulation necessary for adaptation; running faster will jeopardize your chances of successful completion of the next key workout. Furthermore, too fast a pace can lead to overtraining and possible injury.

Q. When should I adjust the paces for faster workouts?

A. You can adjust after running a race that produces a new standard or after you complete all three weekly workouts at the specified paces and feel less than challenged. If either the race time indicates a faster training pace or if all three weekly workout times are easily achieved, then a faster pace should be attempted for the next week's workouts.

Q. Why are there different recovery intervals?

A. The workouts are designed to have a variety of distances and paces. Similarly, the recovery times for repeats are varied. The reason for training at different distances and intensities is that the body adapts when it is pressed to respond to an overload. Different types of overload elicit different physiological responses. The workouts are designed to stimulate the key physiological mechanisms needed for improved running performance. Recovery periods can increase or decrease the stress of the workouts. Varying the stressors—distance, pace, and recovery period—is a mechanism for producing changes in the workload and stimulating physiological adaptations.

Q. How important is a warmup and cooldown?

A. Your likelihood for achieving your target paces in your workouts will be enhanced with a proper warmup. The ideal warmup includes some dynamic stretching and a gradual intensity increase in your warmup running. A cooldown will help to keep you from being stiff and sore later.

Q. What if I don't have a track for Key Run #1?

A. Runners who don't have a track for the repeats designated in Key Run #1 have several options. Find a flat section of road or path that has good footing and is safe for intense running. Measure and mark 400 meters. That will enable you to do most of the workouts. The paved areas around the perimeters of superstore parking lots often provide the needed distance. Another option is to use a GPS to measure the distance run. It can be programmed for distance or time. (See "How to Use a GPS Watch for FIRST Training" later in this chapter.)

Q. Can I run more than three times per week?

A. We have conducted training studies that permitted runners to supplement our basic program with additional runs if they wished. What we found is that most runners chose not to do extra runs after the first few weeks because they found that they could perform the three key workouts better with a day of recovery between workouts. There were no differences in the improvement of those who ran only three days per week compared to those who did supplemental easy runs. For that reason, we designed the **3plus2** program to include the three quality runs and two cross-training workouts. An optional cross-training workout is also permitted.

Most programs include running 5 to 7 days per week and running more than three times per week. But for reasons stated throughout this book, we find that much can be accomplished by running three times per week without the accompanying risks of injury.

The FIRST training program doesn't restrict runners to only three runs per week, but any additional runs must not interfere with achieving the target paces of the three key runs. We have had runners report that they were successful by coupling one or two additional runs with the three key runs prescribed by FIRST. As stated before,

FIRST recommends coupling cross-training workouts with the three Key Runs so as to reduce the likelihood of injury and to provide more quality cardiorespiratory training.

Q. Isn't the FIRST 3plus2 training program low on total training miles?

A. There are many differences in individuals' abilities to tolerate training mileage. These differences are influenced by physiology, anatomy, biomechanics, and years of running experience. Typically, smaller, lighter, and younger runners are able to tolerate more miles. These runners become the elite performers who can run hard, run often, and run long. However, many runners, in particular, aging runners, find that they cannot tolerate high mileage weeks built on 5 to 7 days of running. For them, reducing the number of running days per week is appealing and effective. Runners who have limited time for training, are injured, or who are just looking for a fresh approach to training may find that our program can help them achieve faster performances while fitting their training into a balanced lifestyle. Because the FIRST program is lower on training miles than other traditional running programs, it is attractive to those in the aforementioned categories. However, the FIRST **3plus2** training program is **NOT** lower on training volume. A portion of the weekly total of aerobic training is achieved from aerobic modes of training other than running.

For a ballpark estimate of the number of equivalent miles you add to your training volume with cross-training, divide your total number of cross-training minutes by the average pace—number of minutes per mile or kilometer—you would normally maintain on a run for the number of run-equivalent miles or kilometers. For example, you normally do a 5-mile run at an 8:00/mile pace, but today you did 40 minutes of stationary biking at a comparable level of perceived exertion, then those 40 minutes of biking would equal 5 equivalent miles toward your weekly total training volume.

Q. Will the low mileage program enable me to meet my running goals?

A. Not only is it our belief, but also it is borne out by our own experiences and those of the runners we have trained and the many runners who have followed the FIRST training program that by **Training with Purpose** runners can achieve the high level of fitness necessary to improve running performances. These three runs will require devoting only 3 to 5 hours per week to running. The three sessions per week of high quality running still provide the runner with the fitness benefits of high intensity training and the stimulation, physiological and psychological, associated with hard efforts.

Q. Will my fitness improve more with distance or intensity (speed)?

A. Training volume and intensity are both critical factors in improving fitness. Runners often find it challenging to find the right balance of volume and intensity. If you run a lot of miles each week, it becomes difficult to run at a pace fast enough to stimulate the physiological adaptations needed to get faster. If you run very fast for each run, it is difficult to get the total mileage necessary for building endurance. That's why FIRST has designed and incorporates three key run workouts with different distances and paces to develop a balance of endurance and speed.

Q. How does hill training fit into the 3plus2 training program?

A. The FIRST training program emphasizes the importance of maintaining the proper pace for all key workouts. We understand that the pace for a tempo run and long run will be affected by hills. More time will be lost on the uphills than gained on the downhills, but the two should even out roughly on an out-and-back or loop course. There is no easy rule for adjusting pace times for hills since the steepness, total elevation gain, etc., would have to be calculated.

Try to simulate race course terrain with your training course, if possible. If your planned race is on a hilly course, then train by using hills in longer runs as well as tempo runs. If you live in a flat area you can treat bridges, overpasses, and parking decks as hills to incorporate hill training into your training. Hills certainly add stress to your training. That stress can make you a stronger runner.

Learning to run hills economically takes practice. Obviously, it is tough to run your target paces over rolling, hilly courses. While your average pace over the distance of your run should be near to your target pace, you won't be running a constant pace, but you should be running at a constant effort. Your effort up and down hills should be the same. That means you will run slower than target pace up and faster than target pace down. You need to remain focused on the downhill sections of your running, which is where runners tend to relax. Staying focused on your effort for the duration and distance of your tempo and long runs will translate well to race day.

Stress from hills not only taxes the cardiorespiratory system, it also stresses the muscles and connective tissue. Plantar fasciitis and Achilles tendinitis can develop from excessive hill running. Be sure to stretch the calves before and after hill running. If like a lot of runners you have tight calves, you might need to limit the amount of time spent going up and down.

If you are headed to Boston in April, be sure to include hill training in your preparation. Be prepared to run several miles uphill after miles of long, gradual downhill running that fatigues the quads.

Q. Why is the longest marathon training run only 20 miles?

A. There is no definitive study or theory for determining the optimal distance for the marathon long training run. I know runners who have run very good marathons with no run longer than 15 miles and runners who like to do at least one overdistance (>26 miles) long run. Most marathon programs recommend long runs of 20 miles. Running farther than 20 miles makes it difficult to recover, thus interrupting one's training program. Where the threshold is located that stimulates adaptation and improvement versus the threshold that leads to prolonged fatigue is a mystery. I am sure that it differs by individual, especially with the training pace of the individual. Consider that a 2:40 marathoner will complete a 20-mile training run in a little over 2 hours while a 5:00 marathoner will take 4 hours. Their recoveries from those efforts will be quite different.

We know that most marathoners stick to the 20-mile distance and are able to run excellent races with that preparation. FIRST recommends 20 miles as the longest training run because it is difficult to have a high quality training run (meaning it is difficult to maintain a pace close to marathon pace) at a distance greater than 20 miles. So to run farther than 20 miles most likely will mean that you are running more slowly.

Q. Is it better to run 20 miles near marathon pace or run farther at a slower pace?

A. The FIRST training program is based on pace, and our training philosophy is based on intensity. Intensity is the variable that contributes most to fitness. Thus, we prefer a long run that is faster than what most other programs recommend. That is the most distinctive feature in our training program, along with running fewer days per week with potential additional runs replaced with cross-training.

Q. Why does FIRST recommend five long training runs of 20 miles?

A. Many runners ask, "Why so many?" Others, "Why so few?" There's nothing magical about five or any other number. We have had runners qualify for Boston with only one 20-mile run using our novice marathon program. There is no one training program that is ideal for everyone. However, in general, our experience in both running and coaching is that it's the long runs that best prepare you for the marathon. Too many long runs and your legs become fatigued, too few and you aren't trained to handle the race day pace for the distance. We think five 20-mile runs over 15 weeks provide a good preparation.

Q. Is it okay to enter a race and do my training run?

A. Runners enjoy taking part in races, and so they often ask if it's okay to run one at the target training pace. If the race distance is shorter than their designated training run distance, they say that they will run some additional miles before or after the race. If the race is longer than their designated training run distance, they say that they will drop out once that distance has been completed. In theory, these strategies should work. In practice, they frequently fail to happen as proposed. Too often the runners write after the race that they were feeling good, the pace felt easy, and that they were pulled along by the crowd and finished the race much faster than the targeted training pace or, in the case of the race being longer than their designated training distance, they were feeling good and decided not to drop out. Too often the targeted race and the preparation for it are undermined by using a race for training.

Q. I had a bad training run. What happened?

A. Runners who are following the FIRST training program typically see their fitness improve and their training times get faster. After several weeks of improvement, they write us frantic over a poor training run—much slower than usual, or perhaps they weren't able to complete it. It is common to have a bad run, as it is common to have a bad day. Why? We don't always know, but work, sleep, nutrition, cumulative fatigue, weather, and the unknown are among the factors. Accept it as part of the training cycle and don't worry about it. It happens to everyone.

Q. What am I to do if I miss a workout? A whole week? Multiple weeks?

A. Do not be concerned about a missed workout, nor should you try to squeeze it in later. Stay on schedule with the next workout and don't risk interfering with it. In particular, it's not a problem if you missed the workout because of your personal schedule. It becomes more complicated if you missed a workout because of injury. That's addressed in a later chapter about injuries.

If you miss a week of training, it's typically not a problem, either. Over 16 weeks you aren't going to lose your fitness with missing a week. Again, continue with the schedule as if you had completed that missed week's training.

If you miss 2 or more weeks of training, you need to reconsider your targeted race and determine if your goal should be redirected to another race. It somewhat depends on when those 2 weeks were missed and why. If they were missed in the first 4 weeks of the training program, and you were reasonably fit when you began it, you can most likely continue with the program without concern. If you missed the 2 weeks in the middle or near the completion of the training program, you will need to assess how much fitness was lost. More important is what you were doing those 2 weeks. That is, if you were doing serious cross-training and staying fit that's one thing, but if you were on a cruise just chillin' and likely to have gained several pounds, that's a very different situation. I have heard from folks who reported both of the last two scenarios and my advice was quite different. The former was told to continue with the training program and the latter was told to pick another race as a goal.

Q. Does FIRST recommend training with a heart-rate monitor?

A. FIRST does not use heart rate as a gauge of intensity for its key running workouts. We prefer using pace as a determinant of intensity. Heart rate fluctuations are caused by a variety of variables and do not reflect running speed. A few of those variables, but not an exhaustive list, include body position, core temperature, hydration, emotions, time of day, amount of sleep, recovery status, nutritional status, and medications.

During a long run at a steady pace, your heart rate will increase initially and then level off as the oxygen requirement of the activity is met. However, prolonged exercise at a constant intensity places an increasing load on the heart. Although the metabolic demands of the exercise do not increase, there is a progressive decrease in venous return of blood to the heart. So if venous return drops, there is less blood in the heart and stroke volume (the volume of blood pumped from one ventricle of the heart with each beat) therefore drops. Your heart rate increases to compensate for the reduced stroke volume. The resulting decreased stroke volume and the accompanying increase in heart rate are referred to as cardiovascular drift. This drift is generally due to decreased plasma volume caused by sweating. Thus, if you are maintaining a constant heart rate during that long run, you will gradually run more slowly throughout the run. That won't prepare you to run a constant pace in your next race.

Q. Can FIRST Key Runs be performed on a treadmill?
A. Yes. Many runners do Key Runs #1 and #2 on the treadmill. Most report doing so because they need to run early in the morning or late at night and prefer not to run in the dark. Running in the dark increases the likelihood of an accidental injury, especially if the ground is covered with snow and ice. Beyond reducing the likelihood of an accidental injury, running on the treadmill probably provides a better cardiorespiratory workout than a slower, cautious run on a slick outside surface. In summer, runners from the South report doing their workouts on the treadmill in an air-conditioned space rather than running slowly in extreme heat and humidity.

Our research shows that the oxygen and energy costs for running at the same speed are the same running on the treadmill as compared to running on the road. The treadmill does not need to be adjusted with elevation as long as the treadmill is calibrated accurately. That cannot be assumed. We find that belts on treadmills become loose and do not always travel at the speed that is displayed on the monitor. Runners often contact us for help in translating speed in miles-per-hour to minutes-per-mile. For that reason, we have provided a table in Appendix A that provides those equivalencies.

Q. How do I choose my race pace?
A. For the half-marathon and marathon, your training program designates your HMP (half-marathon pace) and MP (marathon pace) from Table 5.8. That's your race pace. If during the 16-week training program you are able to do all three key runs without pushing yourself, you should use a faster 5K reference time for selecting your training targets and paces from Tables 5.6–5.8. That will result in a faster HMP and MP, which determine your target half-marathon and

marathon target finish times. For the 5K schedules, your target race finish time is determined by your 5K reference time used for selecting training targets and paces. For the 10K target race finish time, refer to Table 2.1 and find the 10K time comparable to your 5K reference time.

Q. What training pace adjustments need to be made at elevation?

A. While the oxygen content of the atmosphere is at a constant percentage (20.9 percent), at higher elevations the atmospheric pressure decreases, reducing the partial pressure of oxygen, which makes less oxygen available for the runner. Endurance activities are hampered at higher elevations beginning at around 3,000 feet. The extent of the performance reduction depends on the distance of the event and to the extent that the individual is acclimatized. The effects of elevation are greater on longer distances. At 5,000 feet, expect a 3.5 percent reduction in performance in a 10K; at 7,500 feet, expect a 6.3 percent reduction in performance in a 10K.

We received a message from three women in Santa Fe, New Mexico, an elevation of 7,000 feet, asking how they could use the FIRST training program for a 3:30 marathon. I knew that they could not expect to run FIRST's target paces designated for the 3:30 marathon, so I suggested that they use the training paces for a 3:38 marathon and that having trained at those paces at elevation, they could run a 3:30 at sea level. All three achieved their 3:30 goals.

HOW TO USE A GPS WATCH FOR FIRST TRAINING

GPS-enabled watches are replacing the traditional chronograph long worn by runners. Runners have been asking us for several years if the FIRST training program is available for their Garmin, the most popular GPS for runners. Fortunately for them, there is Dr. Butch Hill, an electrical engineering professor at Ohio University. Butch is a longtime FIRST training program user. He generously offered to respond to FIRST requests for sharing the Garmin programming for the FIRST key runs. For several years, we have forwarded him those requests. He agreed to provide the following instructions for this edition, so that they are widely available:

Runners of almost any ability can use a Garmin Forerunner effectively for the key runs, because explicit paces and distances for every workout are set in the workout plans and pace tables. The design of the Forerunner employs a similar approach: paces are set in customized "speed zones," and separately entered workouts use those speed zones. When you enter the workouts you can specify the length of each workout element, the target zone for that element, and the rest intervals. There are other workout devices offering similar capabilities, but my familiarity is with the Forerunner.

It is fairly straightforward to set up the FIRST key runs using a Forerunner, together with Garmin's Training Center software. Set your speed zones as specified in Table 5.9, then program the appropriate rest and workout distances.

There are multiple benefits to using a Forerunner for your workouts. You don't need a track to do the workouts, and all your running data are automatically recorded. Once you learn which beeping tone means "speed up," "slow down," and "stop," you don't have to even look at the device during your workout. But there are minor drawbacks, too. There's the temptation to keep looking at the display to see how well you're doing (thereby assuring that you will *not* do as well as you could, as running with your wrist in front of your face doesn't help your form). Batteries can die in the middle of a workout (for those who forget to recharge), or the Forerunner can suddenly lose its GPS fix. Losing the fix can be especially irritating because the device will then assume that you're not moving and hound you to speed up, even if you're going all out! I have an older model and understand that the newer models are less likely to lose the GPS fix.

How to Set Your Forerunner

Table 5.9 gives an overview of the appropriate "My Activities" settings in Garmin Training Center for use with the key runs. Make sure that you set the activity to "Running" for Key Run #1 and to "Biking" or "Other" for half-marathon or marathon training, respectively. You are strongly urged to change the names of the paces from the Garmin defaults to the key run names (e.g., change "Snail," "Turtle," etc., to "Easy," "MP + 60," etc.). For Key Runs #2 and #3, you will have to add a few seconds to the paces given in Tables 5.7 and 5.8 for the "Lower Limit," and add a few seconds to those paces for the "Upper Limit."

Key Run #1 paces will require one additional step: the times given in Table 5.6 are for the given distances, **not** paces in minutes/mile or minutes/kilometer. For example, if your 400M time is 0:01:30 in this table, your pace per mile, which is 1609 meters, would be (1609 meters ÷ 400m) times 1:30, or 6:02/mile. You could therefore set your lower limit for Speed Zone 10 to 6:05 and your upper limit to 6:00. Some of your speed zones may overlap, particularly if you're a fast runner: the Forerunner doesn't seem to care. If you are using your Forerunner in metric mode, then you simply need to adjust the pace to that of 1000M. For example, the 400M time would convert to (1000 ÷ 400) times 1:30 or 2.5 × 1:30 = 3:45 per kilometer.

The speed zones have been chosen so that speed increases with zone number. This can be useful for those occasions when your Garmin keeps signaling you to speed up or slow down. As you run, the Forerunner will display the name of the speed zone that you're in. Assuming that you've followed our suggestion to give the speed zones meaningful names, if you're supposed to be running at 1600-meter pace, but the display says "400M," you know that you're going much too hard.

If you program the distances and rest intervals manually, rather than use the programs available online, you'll need to follow the directions in the Garmin Training Center program; see "Creating a New Workout."

Table 5.9

Garmin Speed Zone Settings for Key Runs

GARMIN SPEED ZONE	KEY RUN #1 (ALL) & #2 & #3 (5K & 10K) ACTIVITY: RUNNING	KEY RUN #2 & #3 (HALF-MARATHON) ACTIVITY: BIKING	KEY RUN #2 & #3 (MARATHON) ACTIVITY: BIKING
1	LT*		Easy
2	MT*		MP + 60
3	ST*		MP + 45
4	2000M	Easy	MP + 30
5	1600M	HMP + 30	MP + 20
6	1200M	HMP + 20	MP + 15
7	1000M	HMP	LT
8	800M	LT	MP
9	600M	MT	MT
10	400M	ST	ST

*Marathoners and half-marathoners do not need to enter the LT (Long Tempo), MT (Mid-Tempo) and ST (Short Tempo) paces here unless they would also sometimes follow the 5K or 10K training plans.

REAL RUNNER REPORT

Dear FIRST team,

I wanted to write to thank you for the research that you've put into the *Run Less, Run Faster* training plan and to let you know that I had a very successful marathon following the plan. Yesterday, I ran a PR of 2:57:49 in the Milwaukee Lakefront Marathon. That bests my previous PR (3:02:55) by more than 5 minutes (in 2003) when I was 27 years old. I'm now 36 and hadn't run a marathon in almost 5 years, but I really wanted to break the 3-hour barrier at least once in my life. I followed the training regimen laid out in the book, missing only a few key runs because of fatigue or a minor injury. I used my bicycle commute to work as the cross-training exercise by modifying my commuting route so I could minimize stopping and match the tempo suggested in the cross-training workouts.

I think the strengthening exercises and drills were a critical element in this program that I haven't incorporated in the past. I held up better in the training and the last miles of the race than I have previously because I was a stronger runner.

Thank you again for doing this research and writing the book.

Sincerely,
Justin Marthaler
Network Administrator
Madison, Wisconsin

REAL RUNNER REPORT

Dear Sirs,

Just a quick note to let you know how delighted I am with your marathon training program. I have been following it since the beginning of this year with the aim of qualifying for Boston. That meant achieving a time of under 3:35 given that I am now 50. My previous best time was 3:42 in Athens in November 2009 (admittedly that was uphill all the way). Other than that, most of my marathons were completed in about or just under 4 hours.

My plan was to get a qualifying time for Boston today at the Rotterdam Marathon, which is over a flat course and has a reputation for being quite fast. In fact, I got my qualifying time 12 weeks into the program in Barcelona with a 3:33, but went ahead and did Rotterdam in 3:30:54!

So, thank you very much for designing a wonderfully successful training program.

Xavier Lewis
Director, Legal and Executive Affairs, EFTA Surveillance Authority
Brussels, Belgium

ESSENTIAL CROSS-TRAINING

The "2" of the **3plus2** Training Program

The FIRST training approach recommends 3 days of running and 2 days of cross-training. Although this approach has fewer days of running than many other running programs, the amount of exercise is similar. While we suggest that runners actually run less, our program does not suggest that they exercise less.

We have received many messages from users of the FIRST program describing how the cross-training component has provided welcome variety to their workouts. Many say they were surprised that adding cross-training made the training week more enjoyable. In addition, they agreed that it enabled them to train harder than going for an easy run and that it helped them recover from the quality key runs.

From our FIRST Learning and Running Retreats held on the Furman University campus, we have observed that most runners previously had not completed the cross-training workouts at the recommended intensity. Typically, each group of Retreat participants finds that the cross-training workouts can also be fatiguing. They learn that the bike and rowing ergometer can be taxing when they are used in a focused workout. They find the same to be true of the pool.

Coauthor Scott Murr likes to say that he is a fit person who runs, rather than a runner who is fit. I suppose that, as physical educators, we are not as singularly focused as are many running coaches and authors. We are concerned about total fitness. We have found that cross-training not only contributes to improved running but also enhances total fitness.

Total fitness is an important concept for runners who want to run for a lifetime. Cross-training provides not only the cardiorespiratory endurance necessary for running success, but also the muscular strength, muscular endurance, and flexibility needed to be a strong and enduring runner over many years. Cross-training also contributes to total fitness by developing the body composition, coordination, and balance that reduce the likelihood of injury.

FIRST prefers non-weight-bearing activities such as swimming, biking, and rowing as cross-training activities to complement the three key runs. In this chapter there is a description of the cross-training activities that are commonly used by our readers. Scott Murr describes how to get the most benefit from each cross-training mode. Capitalizing on his knowledge as a 12-time finisher of Ironman Triathlons, six in Kona, Hawaii, we provide a cross-training program to accompany the three key runs. Combining these two training schedules provides a complete FIRST **3plus2** training program.

CROSS-TRAINING: THE ESSENTIALS

- Cross-training is typically defined as an exercise program that uses several modes of training to develop a specific component of fitness. In the FIRST program, cross-training is intended to enhance aerobic fitness.

- Yoga, Pilates, Cross-Fit, and P90X are NOT considered part of the **3plus2** cross-training approach. We address why later in the chapter.

- Cross-training replaces easy run days (junk mileage).

• Cross-training helps reduce the risk of injuries.

• Cross-training allows for a tremendous volume of central circulatory training without overuse of a particular muscle group.

• Cross-training allows for a greater daily training intensity. Even though the same muscle groups are utilized, they are being used differently.

• Non-weight-bearing cross-training activities give the legs and running muscles a well-deserved break, promoting recovery.

• Cross-training provides variety to the training regimen.

• Cross-training workouts can be based on time rather than distance.

MODES OF CROSS-TRAINING

Cycling

Cycling is a non-weight-bearing, low-impact exercise that develops aerobic fitness while allowing recovery for the legs from the demands of running. It helps develop the quadriceps, which can balance the strengthening of the hamstrings and calves that results from running. Cycling can also increase hip and knee joint flexibility. Because there is no pounding with cycling, runners often recover quickly and it does not interfere too much with the demands of the key runs. Performing intervals on a bike can also help increase leg turnover while running and can contribute to improved running speed. High-power bike intervals work the leg muscles even harder than uphill running, but without the impact of hard running.

Cadence is important. Most runners who cycle tend to "push a big gear" with a low cadence when cycling. Cycling is more beneficial when runners work on quick pedaling at a cadence of 80 to 100 pedal revolutions per minute.

If you choose to bike outdoors as a means of cross-training, you will find that cycling is much more expensive than running. While running in the rain or cold may not be the most fun, most runners are able to run regardless of the weather. Cycling in the rain is no fun and can be quite risky. Cycling outside requires much more time than a comparable stationary bike workout. Although cyclists generally have fewer overuse injuries than runners, when a cyclist has a wreck, the injuries can be serious.

Indoor bike workouts are safer than cycling outside. Indoor bike workouts can be social and fun and do not require expensive equipment. With an indoor bike workout, runners are able to go at their own effort levels while still doing a group workout. Weather is not a factor.

However, there are a couple of drawbacks to indoor bike workouts. Not all stationary bikes have the necessary adjustments to provide a good fit. Also, because of the variety of indoor bikes, you may not be able to duplicate exact workloads and workouts from one brand to another.

Swimming

Many runners who begin swimming do so as the result of a running injury. Swimming is an excellent way to improve overall fitness. It increases upper-body strength and endurance while taking much of the stress off the legs. It stretches the hamstrings and increases ankle flexibility, which may aid running performance. Swimming also allows the body to stay active while recovering from a hard run.

Swimming requires much more technique than running. An unfit skilled swimmer can typically outswim a fit runner lacking technique. Runners need to learn how to swim in a streamlined fashion. Once runners feel comfortable moving through the water, they can then start building endurance. There is no doubt that swimming well requires time, commitment, and focused practice, but swimming is achievable for most runners.

While form and technique are important for running, they are much more so for swimming. Without good swim technique, runners often tire before they are able to get a good cardio workout from swimming. For this reason they do not swim regularly. Swimming can be a great cross-training workout for runners if they will be patient and stick with it.

If you want to incorporate swimming as part of your training, FIRST suggests that, just as with the run, you have a plan for the swim workout. A reasonable goal for a runner would be to stay in the water for 30 minutes and move as much as possible. For example, swim one lap, rest 15 seconds, kick one lap using a kickboard, rest 15 seconds, and repeat this sequence for 30 minutes. You could look at this as an interval workout in the water.

Most runners hate kicking because they feel like they are working hard while making little progress down the pool. Commit yourself to the kicking. You will get better and so will your lower leg and ankle flexibility.

If you do not give up on swimming, you will make quick gains. Just as with your running, set a goal for each workout. For example, the first short range goal might be to swim 400 yards/meters nonstop, gradually increasing your goal to 1500 yards/meters.

TIPS FOR SWIMMING

(these are tips for runners who swim, rather than for competitive swimmers)

• Rather than swim with a fast arm turnover, strive to keep the strokes long and relaxed. Distance per stroke is more important than the number of strokes per minute. Count the number of strokes you take for one length of the pool; try to get your stroke count close to 20 (for a 25-yard pool).

• Develop good breathing technique—remember to exhale completely with your face in the water before rolling your head to the side to breathe. If you find that you are getting out of breath quickly, ask a swim instructor to offer some tips on your swim stroke.

• Since runners are accustomed to using their legs for propulsion, many who start swimming kick too hard. Swimming is primarily an upper-body activity since kicking provides only about 10 percent of the forward propulsion. Many runners kick hard because their kick is inefficient. That's because they have tight and inflexible ankles. Consequently, most runners do not like kick sets. However, kick sets not only help with aerobic fitness but also help improve ankle and lower leg flexibility. Scott insists that the improved ankle flexibility achieved through kicking has helped his running.

Deep Water Running

Deep water running (DWR) means running while submerged neck deep without being able to touch the bottom of the pool. DWR simulates running on land but with no impact and no weight on the joints. DWR is probably the most recommended activity for the injured runner.

TIPS FOR DEEP WATER RUNNING

- Try to simulate normal running style.
- Raise the knees up to about hip height, then push down and slightly backward with the foot.
- Bend the arms in a 90-degree angle and swing them from the shoulder.
- Avoid leaning forward from the waist. Keep the hips in line under the shoulders.
- Keep a loosely closed fist and let the legs move you forward.
- Keep the abs tight to support the back.

A flotation device, such as a water-jogging belt, can be worn; however, use of a flotation belt also reduces the work intensity. DWR uses the same motion as running on land and is the most biomechanically specific form of cross-training for the runner.

Because water is more resistant than air, DWR results in a lower leg turnover or stride cadence. This may be a disadvantage of DWR. Since DWR may "train" a slower neuromuscular firing pattern than typical running, FIRST suggests that DWR be used as a cross-training mode only when the runner is injured.

Rowing

Rowing is a good cross-training choice for runners. Most runners are able to quickly learn the motion required.

Rowing is a total-body, non-weight-bearing exercise. It works both the upper and lower body, taking the major muscles through a wide range of motion, which promotes good flexibility.

Because it is an indoor activity, rowing can be done anytime. Finally, rowing is self-paced, so runners of all abilities can use it to develop fitness.

CROSS-TRAINING: Q AND A

Q. How often should I cross-train?

A. With the three key running workouts, include a minimum of two cross-training workouts per week. The number of cross-training sessions is dependent on the total training volume that is reasonable for your fitness level and available time for training, as well as the amount of running that you are doing. Some runners are able to tolerate and benefit from four or more cross-training workouts per week.

Q. How long should cross-training sessions be?

A. Rather than take a 30- to 45-minute easy run, you can cross-train at a higher intensity for the same duration. When cross-training, base workouts on time rather than distance. Just as with running, you can have short, intense cross-training workouts made of short, high-intensity work intervals interspersed with rest bouts. Or mirror tempo workouts with a hard 20- to 25-minute effort. Or imitate the long run with a 2- to 3-hour moderate-intensity workout.

Q. How do I measure the intensity of cross-training workouts?

A. Many aerobic fitness machines have some built-in measure of work output or speed that you can use to judge your effort. Perceived exertion is also a valid measure of exercise intensity. In other words, a 45-minute spin workout at a moderate cadence with little resistance may be an "easy" workout, while a 30-minute spin workout with a faster cadence and moderate resistance may be a "hard" workout.

For cross-training workouts, we ask runners to use perceived exertion for determining the intensity. It would be very difficult, without knowing an individual's fitness for a specific exercise mode or piece of equipment, to recommend a specific workload—leg strength influences your workload on the bike and swimming technique greatly influences your lap times in the pool. Because heart rates vary for the same perceived effort from one mode to another, we do not use heart rates for determining exercise intensity.

Q. Can I cross-train and run on the same day?

A. Yes. Even though the **3plus2** program designates running and cross-training workouts on separate days, an individual seeking a high volume training regimen can supplement the **3plus2** training program with additional cross-training workouts on running workout days. Although most runners will not be eager to add extra training after the intense FIRST run workouts, cycling or swimming can be good cooldown recovery activities after a run. They can also extend a run workout without extending the time of running-related muscular and connective tissue stresses. So that additional cross-training does not interfere with the key run, we recommend that those who want to cross-train and run on the same day complete their key run first.

Q. What are the best cross-training activities for runners?

A. It is important to choose activities that complement your running. A priority is to give the running muscles a break. Activities such as swimming, rowing, and biking all give good cardiovascular benefits without stressing your lower legs and running musculature. These are non-weight-bearing activities that help give the legs and running muscles a well-deserved break, promoting recovery.

Cross-training is an integral part of the FIRST training approach. It is important that you avoid all-or-nothing thinking. New activities require time before one acquires a feel for the activity. Finally, as with running, it is important to learn the sense of proper pacing for the various modes of cross-training.

Q. Can Cross-Fit, P90X, or similar types of activities be used for cross-training?

A. Cross-Fit, P90X, and other approaches to exercise can be intense workouts that can be beneficial for overall fitness. Some of the exercises used in fitness programs are very technique-dependent, and if your form/technique is not good, you are asking for injury.

Intense, short workouts may not be compatible with a runner's desire to get faster over a long distance. These intense workouts are often shorter than 20 minutes, with the focus primarily on the anaerobic component rather than the aerobic component. Short and intense workouts may not be the best approach for helping a runner get faster for a 10K, half-marathon, or marathon. The FIRST cross-training workouts are intended to further develop aerobic fitness.

Cross-Fit and P90X-type workouts are not optimal cross-training workouts in the FIRST **3plus2** program; however, they may contribute to a runner's muscular strength and endurance (see Chapter 12 on strength training for runners) as long as they are not so muscularly intense that they have a detrimental impact on the next run workout.

Q. Can jump rope be used for cross-training?

A. Jumping rope is a great exercise and is considered a mode of cardiovascular exercise. But FIRST recommends non-weight-bearing activities for cross-training. Jumping rope is not just a weight-bearing exercise; it also tends to stress the lower legs. Runners often need to be cautious about the amount of stress they put on their Achilles tendons, and the gastrocnemius and soleus muscles. Jumping rope is not an acceptable mode of cross-training in the FIRST program.

Q. Is spinning class acceptable for cross-training?

A. Spin classes can be quite challenging. They can be good workouts every now and then. Most spin classes vary considerably in effort during the workout as a result of changes in resistance and spin rate. Spin classes are good because they can force you to work harder than you might otherwise.

Q. Can elliptical machines and stair climbers be used for cross-training?

A. Because they are weight-bearing modes that simulate running (without the pounding), this mode is not recommended for cross-training in the FIRST 3plus2 training program. FIRST promotes cross-training in non-weight-bearing modes in an attempt to give the running muscles a recovery opportunity. Elliptical machines are a viable substitute for running during recovery from certain types of injuries.

If you choose an elliptical cross-trainer or stair climber, for proper use of the equipment and a higher-intensity workout, avoid holding on to the handrails.

Q. Should I taper the cross-training before a race? How much?

A. The goal for a runner is to arrive at the start line of a race healthy, fit, rested, and ready to race. During the week leading up to the race, we recommend that runners reduce their training volume and skip the cross-training.

Q. Does yoga count as cross-training?

A. Yoga does not provide the steady, rhythmic activity that provides the cardiorespiratory training needed for improving aerobic fitness. It definitely offers other benefits, such as flexibility, strength, and core training; however, it is not a substitute for the cross-training recommended in our **3plus2** program.

Q. Does weight training count as cross-training?

A. No. FIRST considers cross-training an aerobic workout without the pounding of the legs, an activity designed to complement high-quality run training.

THE PRINCIPLE OF VARIATION

The variation principle has several meanings. After quality run training, runners should cross-train to give their running muscles a chance to recover. The variation principle also refers to utilizing training cycles to vary the intensity and volume of training to help athletes achieve peak levels of fitness. The variation principle also means that athletes should change their exercises or activities periodically so that they do not overstress a part of the body. Changing activities also helps runners maintain their interest in running.

It may appear that the specificity principle and variation principle are incompatible. The specificity principle states that training must be specific to the desired adaptation and the variation principle seemingly asserts the opposite: train by using a variety of activities. The incompatibility is resolved by the degree to which each principle is followed. More specific training is better to the extent that it can be tolerated, but it can become exceedingly boring and risky. Thus, some variety that involves the same muscle groups is a useful change.

FIRST CROSS-TRAINING WORKOUTS

Below are descriptions of cross-training workouts that will enhance your running. Scott Murr has coached many triathletes and helped many runners use cross-training to complement their training. He has drawn on his own experience as a competitive triathlete from sprint triathlons to the Ironman distance to develop effective training workouts. As we have stressed throughout this book, substituting different modes of aerobic training for running workouts can have multiple benefits—reduced likelihood of an overuse injury, increased recovery time for running muscles, variety in training, and even increased training intensity. Scott's suggested cross-training workouts are in Tables 6.1–6.4.

We provide a progressive cross-training program that accompanies the 5K and 10K running schedules and one that accompanies the half-marathon and marathon running schedules. The cross-training programs give two bike workouts, a rowing workout, and a swimming workout in conjunction with the 16-week run training programs.

Runners should select two cross-training workouts for the corresponding week of their run training. **These workouts complement the three key running workouts and are an integral part of the FIRST program.**

You can repeat a workout twice or you can do a workout of a different mode. Scott recommends that you choose different workouts and different modes for variety. It helps to keep the workouts fresh.

Most runners use cycling as their primary choice for cross-training. Tables 6.1 and 6.3 include two cycling cross-training workouts for each week for the 5K and 10K running schedules and half-marathon and marathon running schedules, respectively. The cross-training workouts for the longer race distances are lengthier.

Tables 6.2 and 6.4 include rowing and swimming workouts for each of the training weeks for the 5K and 10K and half-marathon and marathon running schedules, respectively.

Because there is not a comparable measure of intensity among different types of equipment, we suggest that runners use perceived effort as a reference for cross-training effort level or intensity. The effort levels for the cross-training workouts are described in terms related to your key run efforts.

For example, a cross-training workout labeled as "tempo" would be similar to the perceived effort of a Key Run #2 tempo run. A "hard" effort would be similar to the perceived effort of a Key Run #1 track repeat. An "easy" workout is comparable in effort to a warmup, cooldown, or recovery interval.

Table 6.1

Cycling Workouts for 5K and 10K Training

Easy = effort similar to warmup and cooldown; **Tempo** = effort similar to Key Run #2; **Hard** = effort similar to Key Run #1.

WEEK	CYCLING WORKOUT #1	CYCLING WORKOUT #2
12	10 min easy 8 min tempo 7 min easy	10 min easy 10 min tempo 5 min easy
11	10 min easy 2 × (2 min hard, 2 min easy) 5 min easy	10 min easy 14 min tempo 6 min easy
10	20 min tempo gradually increasing the effort as the workout progresses from 5–20 min	5 min easy 15 min tempo 5 min easy
9	10 min easy; 2 × (1 min hard, 3 min easy); 5 min easy	10 min easy 5 min tempo 5 min easy 5 min hard 5 min easy
8	8 min easy 15 min tempo 7 min easy	10 min easy; 5 × (1 min hard, 4 min easy); 5 min easy
7	10 min easy 10 min tempo 5 min easy 10 min tempo 5 min easy	10 min easy 8 min hard 5 min easy 7 min hard 5 min easy
6	10 min easy 2 × (10 min tempo ½ mile at MP) 5 min easy	25 min tempo gradually increasing the effort as the workout progresses from 5–20 min
5	10 min easy 6 × (1 min hard, 4 min easy) 5 min easy	10 min easy 10 min tempo 10 min easy 5 min hard 5 min easy
4	10 min easy 30 min tempo followed immediately by 10 min easy running	30 min easy
3	10 min easy 30 min tempo 5 min easy	10 min easy; 2 × (2 min tempo, 2 min easy); 5 min easy
2	10 min easy 20 min tempo 10 min easy	30 min easy
Race Week	During the week leading up to your race, you may skip the cross-training. The primary goal is to get to the start line, feeling rested and ready to run your best.	

Table 6.2

Rowing and Swimming Workouts for 5K and 10K Training

Easy = effort similar to warmup and cooldown; **Tempo** = effort similar to Key Run #2; **Hard** = effort similar to Key Run #1.

WEEK	ROWING WORKOUTS	SWIMMING WORKOUTS
12	8 min easy 3 min tempo 3 min easy	20 × (kick 1 length, rest 30 sec), using a kickboard
11	7 min easy 4 min tempo 5 min easy	12 × (swim 1 length, rest 15 sec, kick 1 length, rest 20 sec)
10	5 min easy; 4 × (1 min hard, 1 min easy); 4 min easy	20 × (kick 1 length, rest 20 sec), using a kickboard
9	5 min easy; 2 × (3 min tempo, 1 min easy); 5 min easy	Swim (any stroke) and kick for 20 min nonstop
8	5 min easy 12 min tempo 3 min easy	5 × (kick 2 lengths, rest 15 sec, swim 2 lengths, rest 30 sec)
7	10 min easy 15 min tempo 5 min easy	3 × (1 length fast, 1 length easy; 2 lengths fast, 2 lengths easy; 3 lengths fast, 3 lengths easy; 2 lengths fast, 2 lengths easy; 1 length fast, 1 length easy) with 1 min rest between sets
6	5 min easy 2 min hard, 1 min easy 3 min hard, 1 min easy 4 min hard, 1 min easy 3 min hard, 1 min easy 2 min hard, 3 min easy	5 × (swim 8 lengths immediately followed by kicking 2 lengths) Rest 1 min between sets
5	5 min easy 10 min tempo 5 min easy 10 min tempo 5 min easy	Swim (any stroke) and kick for 25 min nonstop
4	5 min easy; 4 × (3 min hard, Cycle 2 min easy); 5 min easy	10 × (swim 2 lengths, rest 15 sec); kick 4 lengths; 10 × (swim 2 lengths, rest 15 sec)
3	5 min easy warmup; 1 × (4 min hard, 1 min easy); 4 × (1 min hard, 1 min easy); 2 × (3 min hard, 1 min easy); 4 × (1 min hard, 1 min easy); 4 min easy cooldown	Swim 4 lengths easy 3 × (2 lengths easy, 2 lengths fast; 30 sec rest); 6 × (1 length easy, 1 length fast, 15 sec rest)
2	5 min easy 20 min tempo 5 min easy	Kick 4 lengths Swim 20 min Kick 4 lengths
Race Week	During the week leading up to your race, you may skip the cross-training. The primary goal is to get to the start line, feeling rested ready to run your best.	

Table 6.3

Cycling Workouts for Half-Marathon and Marathon Training

Easy = effort similar to warmup and cooldown; **Tempo** = effort similar to Key Run #2; **Hard** = effort similar to Key Run #1.

WEEK	CYCLING WORKOUT #1	CYCLING WORKOUT #2
16	10 min easy 10 min tempo 10 min easy	10 min easy; 3 × (2 min hard, 2 min easy); 10 min easy
15	10 min easy 10 min tempo 2 min easy 3 min hard 5 min easy	10 min easy; 2 × (1 min hard, 3 min easy); 5 min easy
14	10 min easy 20 min tempo 10 min easy	10 min easy; 5 × (1 min hard, 1 min easy); 10 min easy
13	10 min easy 8 min hard 2 min easy 8 min hard 10 min easy	30 min easy
12	10 min easy 30 min tempo	5 min easy; 3 × (5 min tempo, 1 min easy); 5 min easy
11	10 min easy 15 min tempo 5 min easy 10 min tempo 5 min easy	35 min easy
10	10 min easy 20 min tempo 5 min easy 10 min tempo 5 min easy	5 min easy 1 min hard, 1 min easy 2 min hard, 1 min easy 3 min hard, 1 min easy 4 min hard, 1 min easy 3 min hard, 1 min easy 2 min hard, 1 min easy 4 min easy
9	10 min easy; 6 × (2 min hard, 3 min easy); 10 min easy	20 min easy 10 min tempo 10 min easy
8	10 min easy 1 min hard, 1 min easy 2 min hard, 1 min easy 3 min hard, 1 min easy 3 min hard, 1 min easy 2 min hard, 1 min easy 4 min easy	20 min easy 5 min tempo 15 min easy

WEEK	CYCLING WORKOUT #1	CYCLING WORKOUT #2
7	10 min easy 15 min tempo 5 min easy 10 min tempo 5 min easy	10 min easy; 5 × (2 min hard, 3 min easy); 10 min easy
6	8 min easy; 7 × (1 min hard, 2 min easy); 8 min easy	15 min easy 10 min tempo 15 min easy
5	5 min easy 15 min tempo 5 min easy 10 min tempo 10 min easy	10 min easy; 8 × (1 min hard, 4 min easy); 5 min easy
4	10 min easy 20 min tempo 10 min easy	20 min easy 5 min tempo 15 min easy
3	10 min easy 30 min tempo 5 min easy	10 min easy; 3 × (2 min hard, 3 min easy); 10 min easy
2	15 min easy 15 min tempo 5 min hard 10 min easy	10 min easy; 3 × (2 min tempo, 2 min easy); 10 min easy
Race Week	During the week leading up to your race, you may skip the cross-training. The primary goal is to get to the start line, feeling rested and ready to run your best.	

Table 6.4

Rowing and Swimming Workouts for Half-Marathon and Marathon Training

Easy = effort similar to warmup and cooldown; **Tempo** = effort similar to Key Run #2; **Hard** = effort similar to Key Run #1.

WEEK	ROWING WORKOUTS	SWIMMING WORKOUTS
16	8 min easy 10 min tempo 5 min easy	20 × (kick 1 length, rest 30 sec), using a kickboard
15	7 min easy 1 min hard, 1 min easy 2 min hard, 1 min easy 2 min hard, 1 min easy 5 min easy	12 × (swim 1 length, rest 15 sec, kick 1 length, rest 20 sec)
14	10 min easy 10 min tempo 5 min easy	20 × (kick 1 length, rest 20 sec), using a kickboard
13	10 min easy 5 min hard 5 min easy	Swim (any stroke) and kick for 20 min nonstop
12	10 min easy 5 min tempo 5 min hard 5 min easy	5 × (kick 2 lengths, rest 15 sec, swim 2 lengths, rest 30 sec)
11	10 min easy; 5 × (1 min hard, 1 min easy); 5 min easy	5 × (swim 8 lengths immediately followed by kicking 2 lengths) Rest 1 minute between sets
10	5 min easy 1 min hard, 1 min easy 2 min hard, 1 min easy 3 min hard, 1 min easy 4 min hard, 1 min easy 3 min hard, 1 min easy 2 min hard, 1 min easy 4 min easy	3 × (1 length fast, 1 length easy; 2 lengths fast, 2 lengths easy; 3 lengths fast, 3 lengths easy; 2 lengths fast, 2 lengths easy; 1 length fast, 1 length easy) with 1 min rest between sets
9	5 min easy 10 min tempo 3 min easy 10 min tempo 5 min easy	25 min moving nonstop in the water; use a combination of swimming and kicking
8	5 min easy 5 × (3 min hard, 1 min easy) 5 min easy	10 × (swim 2 lengths, rest 15 sec); kick 4 lengths; 10 × (swim 2 lengths, rest 15 sec)
7	5 min easy 10 × (1 min hard, 1 min easy) 4 min easy	Swim 4 lengths easy; 3 × (2 lengths easy, 2 lengths fast, 30 sec rest); 6 × (1 length easy, 1 length fast, 15 sec rest)

WEEK	ROWING WORKOUTS	SWIMMING WORKOUTS
6	5 min easy 6 × (3 min hard, 1 min easy); 5 min easy	Kick 4 lengths Swim 20 min Kick 4 lengths
5	5 min easy 15 min tempo 5 min easy	20 × (kick 1 length, rest 15 sec), using a kickboard Swim 20 lengths nonstop
4	5 min easy 5 min tempo 5 min easy 5 min tempo 5 min easy	Kick 4 lengths Swim 20 min Kick 4 lengths
3	5 min easy warmup; 1 × (4 min hard, 1 min easy); 4 × (1 min hard, 1 min easy); 3 × (2 min hard, 1 min easy); 2 × (3 min hard, 1 min easy); 4 × (1 min hard, 1 min easy); 5 min easy cooldown	3 × (1 length fast, 1 length easy; 2 lengths fast, 2 lengths easy; 3 lengths fast, 3 lengths easy; 2 lengths fast, 2 lengths easy; 1 length fast, 1 length easy) with 1 min rest between sets
2	10 min easy 10 min tempo 5 min easy	10 × (kick 1 length the pool; rest 15 sec), using a kickboard Swim 20 lengths nonstop
Race Week	During the week leading up to your race, you may skip the cross-training. The primary goal is to get to the start line, feeling rested and ready to run your best.	

REAL RUNNER REPORT

I signed up to do the Lakefront Marathon in Milwaukee. The program I was using wasn't working for me and my trainer turned me on to the FIRST training program. Most first-time marathon training programs assume you have no running experience. I had lots of experience, it was just long ago.

After reading your book I started to see that everything was clicking. The program was just like track and cross-country practice. Not only did I have to run a specific workout, but I had to do it in a specific time with a certain amount of recovery. The workouts were intense. Especially in the beginning. Towards the middle of the training I felt like I owned the workout.

How did I do? I ran the first marathon of my life, feeling great, with the pacer at 7:38 pace through the 24th mile and only 30 yards behind through 25. Then I hit the wall and finished in 3:21:06. Missed qualifying for Boston by 7 seconds. I'll get it next time.

Thank you for allowing me to run 28 minutes and 19 seconds faster than my race prediction time based off of a half-marathon that was run just 2 weeks prior to starting with your method. It really works and was fun and challenging at the same time. Mixing up the cross-training also really helped to keep me motivated. I have bought three more copies of the book and gave them to my trainer, my brother, and my best friend. I also continue to share the information on your Web site with anyone I can catch, and thanks to your program, that number keeps getting bigger.

Keep up the good work and thanks again!

Bob Sage, DPM
Podiatrist
Beloit, Wisconsin

CHAPTER 7

REST AND RECOVERY

A basic principle of training is overload. Overload is a planned systematic and progressive increase in training stress in order to improve fitness and/or performance. In other words, train hard and become fatigued, then rest and recover while the body accommodates the need to adapt to an increased workload. Repeating this cycle of overload, fatigue, recovery, and adaptation leads to a fitter and faster runner. However, there is a limit to one's capacity to endure and adapt. The progressive overload must be done gradually.

An overload for runners can mean running farther, more often, or faster. It is important that these stressors be gradually increased separately and care must be taken not to increase multiple stressors simultaneously. In other words, overload only one variable at a time.

Other nontraining stressors can add to your overload. These nontraining stressors include elevation, colds and allergies, poor dietary habits, environmental extremes, travel, stressful work situations, and personal relationships. Pay attention to outside stressors and recognize when it might not be a good time to increase your training load.

Most runners tend to think that more training will make them faster. To a certain extent, that is true. However, crossing one's threshold of tolerance for increased stress will result in fatigue that exceeds the body's ability for adaptation. Highly competitive, goal-oriented runners are vulnerable to the lure of dedicating themselves to incessant training with the expectations of significant performance improvements. Those dedicated efforts can prove to be unproductive.

The key to getting faster is to combine the appropriate amount of quality training with adequate rest and recovery. Increasing the overload at a rate that exceeds the body's adaptation ability causes staleness and even exhaustion. This condition of **overtraining** results in an impaired ability to train and perform. If any component of the training program—frequency, intensity, and duration—is increased too rapidly or if the program does not provide adequate recovery from the increased demands, the runner will suffer from the inability to adapt. Recovery and rest are essential components of a training program.

Runners are told to listen to their bodies. It is important to recognize the signs and symptoms of overtraining early and intervene in the cycle with increased rest before fatigue becomes chronic. Symptoms of overtraining include mood disturbances, irritability, sleep disturbances, increased susceptibility to colds, appetite changes, and a struggle to maintain standard training performances.

We have received hundreds of messages from runners who followed the FIRST training program for 16 weeks exactly as it was intended with remarkable results. They comment that they are now "believers" even though they were skeptical when they adopted the program. Usually, they add that their running friends told them that they would never improve while running less. Prior to having adopted the FIRST program, the runners report that they had run more frequently, but with less intensity and less variation in their paces.

Their success exemplifies the importance of balancing quality training and quality recovery. Many runners have made the common error of trying to gain extra fitness, which upsets the ideal balance of training and recovery. Having made and observed these errors ourselves contributed to our creating the **3plus2** training program.

REST AND RECOVERY: THE ESSENTIALS

• Quality training + quality nutrition + quality rest = quality results.

• Recovery is important and has a place in every training schedule.

• Rest and recovery should be defined in a training program just as the workouts are described.

• Successful runners are those who have recovered the best.

• The rate of recovery is influenced by many factors, which include age, fitness level, life stressors, health level, diet, sleep, and exercise background/experience.

• A prerace rest period needs to be planned and must be structured in order to be effective.

• Recovery is vital after a key workout or a race.

• Just as runners taper prior to racing, they should return gradually to quality training during postrace recovery.

• Daily physical activities should be recorded, including rest and recovery activities.

REST AND RECOVERY: Q AND A

Q. When is it important to rest and recover?
A. Once you have completed a key workout or a race, it is important to recover from that training stimulus. The FIRST training approach balances rest and recovery with the quality runs. The day following a key run workout is intended to be a rest day for the weight-bearing running muscles. The idea is to allow the legs a chance to recover so that the next key run can be a quality and productive run.

Q. What can be done to enhance recovery?
A. We mentioned in Chapter 5 that a cooldown after the key runs will aid in preventing soreness and stiffness. We also recommend postworkout static stretching. Many runners say that doing yoga or Pilates helps them recover. Try getting a massage or using a foam roller for relief from muscular tightness.

Q. How should recovery be structured before a race?

A. If you are training for an important race, you must allow your body to recover beforehand. You cannot maintain your normal training and then go straight into a race and expect to run a PR.

Prerace rest does not necessarily mean just 1 or 2 days without running or exercise before race day. A prerace rest period must be significant and must be structured. In a structured training schedule, training builds up gradually (with built-in recovery periods) until some specified period before the target race when the training load usually peaks. Then a taper begins with a reduced training load, usually 2 weeks before a marathon and 1 week before a 5K or 10K. This taper allows the body to recover completely. Then the athlete is fully prepared to race and can reasonably expect to perform at or near his or her best. All FIRST training programs include a taper prior to a race.

Q. How should postrace recovery be structured?

A. Once you have completed a race, it is important to recover from that stress. Improvement occurs during the recovery phase and not the workout itself. The rate of recovery is influenced by many factors. One key recovery factor is postrun hydration/nutrition. (See Chapter 11 on nutrition for postexercise/race recommendations.)

After a race, take a complete rest from running (anything from 2 or 3 days for a 10K to a week or more for a marathon). This is a good time to cross-train. You can stay active yet minimize any additional stress to the primary running muscles. The return to training should be gradual.

Postrace Recovery Guidelines

5K Race: Substitute an easy run for Key Run #1 (Track Repeats) the following week. If your energy levels have returned to normal, then resume normal training with Key Run #2 (Tempo Run). Continue with your normal cross-training. Reduce the intensity if you are experiencing postrace fatigue.

10K Race: Same as post-5K race. In addition, reduce the intensity of Key Run #2 to 90 percent of your normal effort.

Half-Marathon: If you raced an all-out effort, then reduce the intensity of your workouts for the next 2 weeks. Rest the day after the race. Resume cross-training but substitute easy runs for Key Runs #1 and #2 the week after the race. One week later, make the long run half of your normal distance and run at an easy pace. The second week after the half-marathon, resume regular training if you feel rested and have no lingering muscle or joint aches.

Marathon: After a marathon, you need to take a week off from running. YES, we mean it! Follow the week off with a week of easy running, and the third week begin doing your workouts, but at no more than 90 percent effort. If you have no aches and pains after 3 weeks, then you can return to regular workouts.

REAL RUNNER REPORT

Dear Bill and Scott,

I just wanted to tell you that I just ran a marathon PR and qualified for Boston thanks to the FIRST program. In January, some friends convinced me to run the Lincoln Marathon. I had sworn I would never run this particular marathon again . . . but the head of our running group—Team Lizzie—wanted some of us to run the marathon in honor of her daughter (Lizzie) who would have graduated from high school this year.

My friend Laura insisted that we use your FIRST program, which we found in a Runner's World article.

Anyway, I couldn't turn this offer down and I had 5 leftover baby pounds to lose. But I really didn't think I could touch the success stories described in the article.

This was my fourth marathon—my previous times were 4:20 (2006), 4:15 (2007), and 4:16 (2008). Two weeks before the 2008 marathon, I was attacked by a homeless man during a training run, so this sort of derailed any hopes of a PR for that race. And then I had a baby last summer.

This past weekend, not quite 10 months after having my third child, I ran the Lincoln Marathon with a time of 3:37:38!!! What a joy: a PR, a sub-4:00, and a Boston qualifying time (at 35)!!! So thank you, thank you, thank you!!! I loved every minute of the training and will definitely use it again for future marathons!

Nancy Foster, Ph.D.
Assistant Professor
Licensed Psychologist
Munroe-Meyer Institute/University of Nebraska Medical Center
Omaha, Nebraska

(continued on page 116)

FOLLOW-UP MESSAGE:

Hi Bill –

I look forward to continuing to use your training plans. I just ran Boston last week and had a PR of 3:36:04—using your training program for the second time! I just adjusted the times based on my new faster base. My next goal is a 3:30 marathon. I am certain that I can accomplish this with your training program. I continue to enjoy the three (very) hard days of running—it fits neatly into my busy life and makes racing more exciting! At least five of my friends have also converted to using one of your plans!

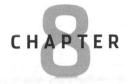

CHAPTER 8

YEAR-ROUND TRAINING

We get a lot of emails from runners asking:

1. How do I train between marathons that are less than 8 weeks apart?

2. Is it okay to run a half-marathon 3 weeks before a marathon?

3. Can a 10K be substituted for a long training run?

Clearly, many runners want to race often, even when it jeopardizes optimal performances. As runners, we understand the interest in racing often. However, it is difficult to achieve peak performance when you race frequently.

At our public lectures, runners bemoan their poor race performances and want to know why. When questioned, they begin listing all of their recent races. I ask them why they run so many races. It's often because they have a favorite race they do every year; they want to accompany friends to a race; they had a bad race and want to vindicate their recent poor performance; or they think they can win an age-group award. I find it difficult to persuade runners to choose a race schedule for the year—one that permits serious training for just a few key races. If you care about optimizing performance, being selective about the races you run is smart.

I find that spring is a good time to focus on a couple of 5Ks and/or 10Ks and incorporate shorter track repeats and faster tempo runs. Maybe even a half-marathon. Fall provides lots of choices for marathons and usually ideal weather for long training runs. Similarly, there are marathons in the spring and shorter races in the fall. The point is that each season needs a particular focus.

You need to be flexible. We suggest that you identify two to four key races a year and then focus on training for them. Low-priority races typically do not fit well into a planned training schedule. I have runners tell me that they are going to run their favorite 10K in April, even though they are training for Boston. By racing a week or two before Boston, they jeopardize their Boston performance, or by racing the following weekend, they invite injury. Year-round training needs year-round planning.

Marathon training is stressful, even with our method that emphasizes recovery, so be cautious about jumping right back into the next marathon training cycle. After the postmarathon recovery month, we recommend 1 to 2 months of lighter training before beginning the next 16-week marathon training preparation. Beginning the marathon preparation too soon after an all-out marathon effort is pushing the limits of what we believe to be prudent and ideal. The time off provides a break from the mental stress associated with the marathon preparation. It is also a good time to run a shorter race and capitalize on the strong base built for the marathon.

We receive a lot of inquiries about how much time is needed between marathons. This question is one of the toughest to answer because there are many factors that enter into the equation. Some individuals recover more rapidly than others. The differences in recovery are influenced by the intensity of the effort and the weather conditions—running in warm conditions when a lot of fluids were lost slows recovery.

We are aware of individuals who have run marathons every week of the year. One runner who contacted us had run marathons for more than 50 months consecutively. In all sports, there are individuals who have special abilities. These individuals may have special recovery capabilities. However, their constant racing may prevent their attaining an optimal performance.

For most individuals, we believe that running more than two marathons per year risks their being overtrained and injured; it also jeopardizes the proper preparation needed for a solid performance. We realize that sometimes runners enter a marathon with the attitude that it is a long training run. However, a marathon is still 26.2 miles of running. Even if you don't run as fast as you are capable of, you'll still need to recover from the biomechanical stress.

YEAR-ROUND TRAINING: THE ESSENTIALS

- For optimal performances, develop a year-round training and racing plan.
- Choose races in advance and develop a training schedule for each race.
- Include a variety of racing distances.
- Develop a plan that includes a variety of training periods.
- Follow a 12-week training schedule for 5Ks and 10Ks.
- Follow a 16-week training schedule for half-marathons and marathons.
- Build in recovery periods after races.
- Target no more than two marathons per year.

YEAR-ROUND TRAINING: Q AND A

Q. Should I train the same way all year long?

A. High school, collegiate, and elite runners have distinct running seasons. High school and collegiate competitors run cross-country in the fall, indoor track in the winter, outdoor track in the spring, and base training in the summer. Elite runners do the summer European track circuit and often a fall or spring road race, which means a major marathon for the long-distance runners. Thus, these competitors have specific training schedules geared toward three or four annual peak performances. Conventional wisdom from exercise physiologists and elite coaches over the past 50 years suggests that training for these peak performances should be divided into distinct training periods, typically referred to as periodization.

Q. How can the age-group runner have training phases compatible with racing goals?

A. The year can be divided into cycles for one key race or up to four key races, one in each season. Race distances should allow ample time for recovery before the next cycle begins. FIRST does not recommend a four-race year that would include all marathons or even a combination of marathons and half-marathons.

Q. What is an example of a year-round racing plan that incorporates different training phases?

A. A training plan that includes a winter 5K, spring 10K, a late summer or early fall half-marathon and a fall marathon provides different types of training that stimulate the physiological adaptations that determine running performance. Training programs must produce the appropriate stimulation to produce workload adaptation. That is, for the 5K there must be more emphasis on intensity for shorter distances and for the marathon more emphasis on endurance.

If a marathon is in your year-long plan, consider that a 16-week training plan, in addition to 2 to 4 weeks of recovery, covers 5 months.

Q. How can the FIRST three-quality-runs per week model be used for a year-round racing plan?

A. The three basic workouts—track repeats, tempo and long runs—can be used year-round as the basic training plan. You will notice that the training plans outlined in Chapter 5 are similar in structure, but the training distances are modified according to the race distance. Running the track repeats and tempo runs at a slightly faster pace is more useful if you are preparing for a 5K and/or 10K; running the long runs at a slightly faster pace is key for half-marathon and marathon training.

Q. How should I train when I am not following one of the FIRST training programs?

A. We use the **3plus2** training program year-round. In between the 12- or 16-week training programs, we still recommend doing an interval workout (Key Run #1), a tempo run (Key Run #2) and a long run (Key Run #3) to maintain fitness and to prepare for the next focused program. For variety, but to keep your training structured, you can do the following:

1. For Key Run #1, go to Tables 5.1–5.5 and choose "track repeats" workouts. You can make up a mixture of these. Another option is to go to our Web site (www.furmanfirst.com) and do the workouts that are posted under Tuesday Track Workouts.

2. For Key Run #2, do a 30- to 45-minute run with at least 15 to 35 minutes at a comfortably hard pace.

3. For Key Run #3, run between 10 and 15 miles if you are a half- or full marathoner or 6 to 8 miles if you are a 5K or 10K racer, so that you maintain your endurance and will be prepared to begin any of the training programs.

While you are doing similar workouts to what you will be doing in one of the FIRST training programs, the off-season training does not need to be as focused on pacing. You should rely more on perceived exertion. You can leave the watch at home. That is, you will give a good effort, but you won't have to worry about hitting the target paces that are an integral part of the FIRST training programs. The same advice can be applied to the cross-training. Choose different modes and enjoy the variety of workouts.

Q. What are the benefits of a training plan?

A. A training plan makes it easier to select your workouts. No matter what training schedule you are following, your plan will detail your workout. You will not have to think about planning a workout when you step on the track or pavement, since you will already have a plan. Having a structured plan has been one of the aspects of the FIRST Training Programs that runners have most enjoyed.

Just as in any planning, adjustments may be needed at times due to injury, illness, fitness level, or other uncontrollable variables. The occasional adjustment to a plan, however, is far simpler than the deciding about each training session when you don't have a plan.

Q. Is it ever acceptable to do marathons back to back?

A. Frequently, we get messages or calls from runners asking how to train for a marathon 4 to 8 weeks after a marathon that they just finished. As noted above, we don't recommend running marathons so close together because you aren't going to get fitter, you are increasing the risk for injury, and you won't recover enough from the marathon just completed. That said, there are times that it might be reasonable to try to get two marathons for the training of one. I worry about saying that because I don't want readers to take that as an endorsement for trying to piggyback marathons.

When is it okay to try a second marathon a short time after the first one? Perhaps, for whatever reason, you weren't feeling right, so you ran at training pace or more slowly. As a result, even though your performance was subpar, your recovery from the less taxing effort was immediate, similar to a training run. The same could happen if race-day conditions were difficult (think the heat and humidity at Chicago 2007) and you were smart, didn't run at planned marathon pace, but instead ran prudently around the city and collected your finisher's medal. In each of those cases, it would be reasonable to consider another marathon in the next two months.

Depending on the level of stress and/or fatigue the marathon caused, you could resume training in a couple of days, and if there is another marathon within the next 4 weeks, you could plan one more long run of 15 miles and then follow the last few weeks of the marathon training plan in Table 5.5. Yes, you would have two tapers for your training plan. But you have to figure that the 26.2-mile race, even if it was run at slower than race pace, was probably more stressful than what you are willing to admit. It would be wise not to try to squeeze any extra hard work in for that next marathon.

If your second marathon is 2 months away, then you could resume the marathon training plan starting at week 7 or 6 and follow it to the end.

Note: If you ran a hard effort that ended with a disappointing finish time, we do NOT recommend you run another marathon right away. Even though there is an urge to redeem yourself immediately, your disappointment in almost every case becomes greater. Take a month to recover and then target another marathon several months away. With marathons filling so fast, planning for many of them must be done months in advance.

COMMENTS ON SHORT- AND LONG-TERM PLANNING

Runners benefit from a training plan, both short-term and long-term. Having a plan that outlines training and racing for the coming year increases the likelihood that a training schedule with different emphases is included. A variety of training is necessary to stimulate the physiological responses needed for adaptations.

A training plan helps ensure that a runner follows a structured program. Breaking the training process into phases with specified workouts over well-defined periods provides identified targets. These targets serve as training goals. These training goals can be used to give the runner a measure of accountability.

REAL RUNNER REPORT

Hello Dr. Pierce,

I bought your book in the spring and used the FIRST program to train for my first marathon, the Prince Edward County Marathon. A couple of months ago, you very kindly and promptly gave me some email advice about tapering with cycling and strength training. Your program made so much sense to me that, training completely on my own, I followed it as closely as possible. I never had the slightest hint of injury. I especially took to heart your advice about even pacing.

I am 56, female. I needed to finish in 4:15 to qualify for Boston. My chip time was 4:09:52, pace 5:55/K. I ran the first 21K in 1:25:38, a pace of 5:59/K. I ran the next 21.195K in 1:24:15, pace 5:52. I ran the last 5.195K in 5:40, and the last 1.195K in 5:24 . . . it was great to finish feeling so strong.

Thanks to your program, I plan to visit Boston in the spring!

Merci beaucoup!

Shirley Donald, M.D.
Anesthesiologist
Orillia, Ontario, Canada

FOLLOW-UP MESSAGE:

You will be glad to know I did run Boston last year and had a fabulous time. I ran it in negative splits and requalified. However, I decided to make it a once-in-a-lifetime event. I actually just took your book off the shelf this week, in view of seeing whether I can qualify for the NYC Marathon.

SECTION III
Performance Factors

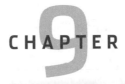
RUNNING HOT AND COLD

As any experienced runner knows, the weather is a critical race performance factor. Months of excellent training can easily be undermined by high temperatures or humidity, a chilling headwind, or subfreezing temperatures. Before selecting a race, I check the 10-year weather history for the race city. As any runner soon finds out, averages can indicate only the likely temperature for a specific day. You make your race choice and hope that playing the percentages pays off.

What do you do on those days that the unexpected occurs and the conditions are extreme? You have the choice of not running the race and choosing another within the next couple of weeks. That choice will give you a chance to perform in conditions that are more conducive to achieving the goal finish time representative of your months of training. Another choice is to run the race because it is one that you particularly want to experience. It may also be likely that you have incurred travel expenses and made arrangements with friends to share the race experience. For whatever the reason, you must modify your goal finish time and your planned race pace, realizing that the conditions dictate the modification. The worst choice is to believe that you can defy conditions and successfully run to your potential against the heat, wind, or extreme cold.

We receive many messages from runners in the southeastern United States or Southeast Asia asking how to train in heat and humidity. In the western part of the country, the low humidity and large daily range of temperature provide cooler times of day for workouts. However, in the regions of the country with high humidity, it is not possible to run as fast in the summer months. So how should runners in these regions adjust their summer running?

There's no question that heat and humidity will slow your pace. This poses a problem for the runner who is using the summer months to prepare for a fall race. Because you will most likely not be running your fall marathon in the extreme heat and humidity that you will experience in the summer, training in very high temperatures that cause you to run 30 seconds per mile slower than your normal training pace will not provide the preparation needed for that fall race.

To combat this problem, we prepare during the summer for fall marathons by running early in the morning when the temperatures are typically in the low 70s with little radiant heat, even though the humidity is high. There will still be a performance decrement, but the neuromuscular and biomechanical training will not be much different from fall training and racing. You can expect to run a little slower than your normal targeted pace. As long as your effort is challenging but doable, you will be getting the benefits you are seeking. Running in the afternoons with a 90+ degree heat index does not permit the faster running needed for training specificity, at least not safely.

We recognize that our location in the western part of the Carolinas provides cooler temperatures than those near the coast or those in the Deep South, where temperatures can be in the 80s or even 90s in early morning. For those runners, it makes sense to choose a late fall race so that there is time to perform long training runs in early fall with cooler temperatures. In Chapter 5, we discussed using a treadmill for performing runs at a faster pace than what is possible outside. The lower temperature and humidity of the indoor environment will enable you to run at a faster pace than the outdoor heat would permit. Mixing outdoor running for acclimatization with indoor running for speed may be a good race preparation strategy. Consider the specificity principle. Try to train in conditions similar to those you will be racing in.

THE ESSENTIALS: RUNNING HOT AND COLD

• Ideal conditions for running performance is 40° to 60°F (5° to 16°C) and low humidity.

• Heat and cold above and below the ideal have adverse effects on running times.

• Heat is the most dangerous and most difficult environmental condition to combat.

• Properly hydrate before, during, and after workouts in hot conditions.

• Avoid comparing training and racing times run in the heat to times run in ideal conditions.

• Reduce exercise intensity in very hot conditions.

• During hot weather, train in the early morning when the temperatures are coolest.

• Acclimatize to heat for 7 to 14 days when warm weather begins.

• The adverse effects of cold can be minimized with proper clothing and apparel accessories.

RUNNING HOT AND COLD: Q & A

Q. What is a hot environment?

A. When the temperature begins to climb over 60°F (16°C), you can expect the temperature to influence your running, i.e., 1 to 2 percent loss of running economy for each 1.5°F increase in temperature. This performance decrement becomes more pronounced as the race distance increases. Add increased humidity to an already warm day and the impact is even greater. Your expected performance goals must be adjusted when you encounter high temperatures and humidity.

Q. How important is hydration in countering the effects of heat?

A. Very important. The answer to this question could easily be an entire chapter. You must be aware that hydration becomes a key factor in running performance in those sessions lasting more than 1 hour. A 2 to 3 percent water loss will result in a significant performance decrement.

Q. How can you be sure you are drinking enough but not too much?

A. Make sure that your urine output is plentiful and the color clear or pale yellow before you begin running. If you lose more than 2 percent of your body weight during a run, you need to drink to avert a compromised performance.

Q. How do you acclimatize to the heat?

A. Heat acclimatization requires exercising in the heat. Sitting in a hot environment, even for extended periods of time, will not result in the adaptations necessary for exercising in the heat. The body learns to sweat more effectively and to tolerate liquid replacement as it trains in hot environments. The body requires 10 to 14 days for complete acclimatization to elevated environmental temperatures, although initial adaptations occur in the first 5 days of acclimatization.

Q. What's a runner to do when it's hot?

A. You will not be able to sustain as fast a pace as normal in the heat, even after adequate acclimatization. In Key Run #1, you may substitute short repeats (400s, 800s) for longer repeats (1200s, 1600s). Another strategy is to take longer recoveries between repeats and hydrate throughout the workout. In Key Runs #2 and #3, you may not be able to maintain the prescribed pace for the specified distance. Run at an effort you perceive as moderate to hard. When running in hot, humid conditions, be smart and listen to your body.

Q. How do I know if I am encountering a heat disorder and what should I do?

A. There are three major categories of heat injury: heat cramps, heat exhaustion, and heatstroke. Heat exhaustion is the most common type of heat injury experienced during running competitions. All of these conditions can be prevented with proper fluid intake and by paying appropriate attention to the symptoms associated with heat disorders—headaches, excessive sweating or cessation of sweating, muscle spasms, irritability, and disorientation. Heat injuries can be serious. It is important to stay hydrated, listen to your body, and train smart. It's not necessary to risk your health to complete a run just because it's on your schedule.

Q. What are the risks associated with exercising in the cold?

A. Exercise in cold environments presents few risks to the runner who makes proper preparation. The runner must pay close attention to dress, hydration, length of race, and energy sources. As long as you generate more heat than you lose, exercising in the cold should not present the problems that exercising in the heat does.

Q. How should the runner dress for cold weather?

A. We wish we could create easy-to-use tables for choosing racing gear for every 10-degree interval. However, while many runners are comfortable in a short-sleeved T-shirt at 40 degrees, some want a long-sleeved shirt any time the temperature drops below 50 degrees.

Even with the wide variation in individuals' toleration of cold, there are some general guidelines we find useful. The most important is to remain dry while keeping warm. Adding layers of clothing as the temperature drops and/or the wind picks up is usually the most effective way to keep moisture away from your body. The layer next to your body should be a material that wicks moisture from your skin. Silk will accomplish that, as will a number of high-tech synthetic materials. Even when you are wearing only a T-shirt, it's a good idea to keep the moisture away from your skin. Remember—you perspire constantly and the rate of sweating increases as you exercise harder.

You may need to add a second layer of insulating material such as wool, down, or fleece if you need to keep body heat in. Finally, if you are running in severe conditions, you may need to add a wind- and water-resistant shell to protect you from the elements. This layer should be capable of letting moisture pass outward. The advantage to using layering is that you can peel off unneeded clothing if conditions improve or if your body provides sufficient heat to keep you feeling warm.

Once the temperature is below freezing and especially if it's windy, you must guard against frostbite. Gloves are fine, but mittens conserve more heat. Remember to cover your head, since a great deal of heat is lost through the head. Finally, socks that wick moisture are just as important for cold-weather running as they are for hot-weather running. Your feet produce great amounts of moisture that need to be eliminated. Breathable shoes will complement high-tech wicking socks.

Q. Is hydration important in cold weather?

A. Most individuals tend to take in less liquid in the cold, even when exercising. Just as in the heat, thirst is a very poor measure of your need for fluids. Fluid replacement in a cold environment is important, but the need typically is not as obvious to the runner as it is in warm conditions.

Q. What's a runner to do when it is cold?

A. Follow the guidelines above and be prepared to be uncomfortably cold for the first 10 minutes of your run. If you are comfortable when you start your run in the cold, you will be too hot once you begin producing heat. It is well worth the expense of purchasing technical clothing that wicks away moisture. You can remain remarkably dry while running. Having dry clothes makes all the difference for staying warm and enjoying a winter run.

When checking the temperature to determine how many layers to wear, pay attention to the windchill factor. Wind can reduce the effective temperature considerably. It is nice to have an outer layer that can be zipped and unzipped as you move into a headwind or a tailwind. And don't forget the sunscreen just because it's cold!

REAL RUNNER REPORT

Dear FIRST program,

I am 31 years old and have been running since 2004. I started out walking, and then completed my first marathon in October of 2004 with a time of 4:58. Since then, I have completed seven more, most recently, the Medtronic Twin Cities Marathon, which I did yesterday. I had been one of the runners you discuss in your book, *Run Less, Run Faster,* who ran to get in miles, but had no real purpose for WHY I was running the distances or paces that I did.

Qualifying for Boston is a goal for me, but my fastest marathon was in 2006 at 4:10. My age- group requires a 3:40 to qualify, which until yesterday seemed out of the realm of possibility. I took a look at your program for a couple of reasons. First, I had always "heard" of speedwork, but had no idea what it entailed; how fast to go, for how long, with what recovery? Secondly, being part of a newly blended family with three children instead of one, I needed to be home with my family more. Your program allowed that.

Using your program, I had trained to run a 3:53 marathon which I chose based off a recent 24:00 5K time. I had run a 1:51 half-marathon in May of this year, but to be honest, I felt that the 3:53 marathon was pushing it. The FIRST program was great. I got all my workouts in and felt refreshed, not exhausted at the beginning of each. I didn't dread the runs, like I typically do when I was running 40+ junk miles a week just to get in "my mileage." I lost over 10 pounds and am significantly quicker now than before.

Yesterday, at the Twin Cities Marathon, I ran a PR chip time of 3:49. I was on pace to qualify for Boston until mile 21, where I hit some large hills and felt my entire energy supply disappear. While I am pleased that I cut 21 minutes off my prior fastest time, I am unsure of how to train for those last 5 miles, or what I could have/should have done differently. I'm happy to provide any additional information about myself if it would be helpful. I'll make a solid attempt at a BQ time next fall on a fast, flat course and I will use the FIRST plan. I recommend it to everyone I know, and I will never be a "junk mileage" runner again. Thank you!

Emily J. Blomme
Quality Assurance Director
Horizons, A Family Service Alliance
Cedar Rapids, Iowa

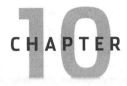

CHAPTER

RUNNING INJURIES

It is common for FIRST to receive messages from runners describing a recent injury and asking what to do about their training for an upcoming race. I don't hesitate, based on my experiences both as a runner and coach, to urge runners to stop running and get an evaluation of the injury from a health professional, preferably a physical therapist who is familiar with running injury treatment. Treating soreness or injury symptoms early diminishes the length of the recovery and the time missed from running. Early intervention can also reduce the likelihood of an injury becoming serious.

Unfortunately, runners are often in denial about an injury. Or they may recognize it and hope that they can "run through it." Sometimes you can, but it's rare. Continuing to train with an irritation usually means that the inflammation worsens. More than one runner has written me stating that they are nearing the end of a long preparation for an important race and that "taking time off now is not an option." More likely than not, that runner will write me several weeks later saying that he or she can no longer run and that it hurts even to walk. At some point during their running lives, most people will have to face a decision of whether to continue training or to stop and heal.

Like many runners, I have suffered miserably with plantar fasciitis and Achilles tendinitis because I kept training through the soreness and pain. Both injuries are devilish to eliminate, especially when you continue training after detecting the symptoms. The more inflamed the tissue, the longer the recovery. Now I take preventive and rehabilitative measures at the first hint of an irritation. With an appropriate training program and a conservative approach to irritations, downtime from running can be kept to a minimum.

Pay close attention to your body and keep it in good shape. A physical therapist or chiropractor would recommend stretches and strength training to address poor flexibility and muscular weaknesses after you are injured. We advocate doing stretches and strength training as **prehab** rather than **rehab**. The flexibility and strength training exercises and form drills that we include in this book can be done in a reasonable amount of time and not only will improve performance but will provide a good defense against injury.

Many runners have reported that reducing the number of days and miles has been the answer to addressing their injuries. By eliminating the injuries, these runners are able to train with the intensity needed to improve their fitness and running performance. It is gratifying that the FIRST program is enabling runners to pursue and achieve running goals that, because of previous injuries, they thought no longer attainable.

We have found it difficult to convince people to reduce their running as soon as they incur an irritation, regardless of the statistical evidence we present. When runners contact us about an injury and we ask how long they've been having problems, the answer is often "months." We insist that runners we coach inform us as soon as they recognize any symptom of injury. We immediately have them reduce their distance and pace. If that doesn't help to relieve the problem, we reduce the frequency of running. We also suggest other conservative treatments, such as ice, massage, ultrasound, stretching and strengthening, and nonsteroidal anti-inflammatories. By insisting that these guidelines be followed, we have been able to help runners continue their training with only minor modifications, rather than a significant training interruption.

Below we answer commonly asked questions about injuries and describe in some detail the most common running injuries, the causes, the signs and symptoms, and the treatments.

RUNNING INJURIES: THE ESSENTIALS

• Most runners will incur an injury at some point that will interfere with their training.

• The majority of these injuries will be associated with the anatomy at or below the knee.

• The majority of running injuries are related to doing too much too fast or too soon.

• Training should be modified until the injuries have mended.

• The sooner and more aggressively injuries are treated, the sooner they will be repaired.

RUNNING INJURIES: Q AND A

Q. What are acute injuries?

A. Strains, partial tears of muscle and sprains, partial tears of ligaments and tendons are classified as acute injuries and usually occur as a result of a fall, twisting movement, or a forceful, explosive movement, such as jumping and sprinting. The immediate application of compression, ice, and elevation of the injured area will reduce the inflammation and swelling. Seek medical help, if the pain or swelling is severe. Rest the affected part until pain and swelling are greatly reduced or absent. Begin a return to activity by strengthening the injured area, followed by a gradual return to full activity.

An injury does not necessarily preclude activity altogether. You may be able to bike or swim depending on the specific location of the injury.

Q. What are overuse injuries?

A. Overuse injuries are chronic orthopedic irritations resulting from repetitive strain on a body part. Running contributes to repetitive stress on muscles, tendons, and bones. Without adequate recovery, overuse injuries can develop. The body can recover from most of this stress, but only if it has adequate time for the tissue to adapt, compensate, and strengthen. Just how fast the adaptation occurs is related to age, overall condition, and the gradual progression of increased training.

Q. How much running is too much?

A. This question is not easily answered. There is a wide range among individuals as to their tolerance for running frequency and duration—two primary factors that determine overall stress. Adding days of running must be balanced against the increased likelihood of injury. The length of runs must be gradually increased. Too much, too often, leads to injury.

Q. Is training intensity associated with injuries?

A. Intense training is a fundamental part of the FIRST approach. Intensity brings the greatest gains in performance, but presents the risk of injury. How to balance the use of intensity with the prevention of overuse injuries is one of the challenges that all runners face. The intensity (pace) must be gradually increased. Just because you are capable of running faster doesn't mean that you should be doing so in each workout.

Increased intensity or running faster for the workout should not be added while also increasing distance. Manipulate only one of the three primary training variables—frequency, duration, and intensity—at a time.

In particular, be careful with track repeats if you are not accustomed to that type of intense training. Running fast provides many cardiorespiratory benefits, but it also changes running form, and for some that can mean transferring the stress to a different set of muscles.

Q. How can overuse injuries be prevented?

A. To prevent overuse injuries the runner needs a prudent, well-defined program of running. The design of FIRST's three-days-a-week program is ideal for runners who may be injury-prone. Elite runners who are willing to bear the risks of injury associated with greater intensity, frequency, and duration of effort are not likely to find our approach appealing. For the average competitive runner, the costs of pushing to the limits, as measured in injuries and lost training days, are not likely to be worth the marginal improvements.

Q. How do I know if I have a biomechanical or anatomical problem?

A. These two categories are not mutually exclusive, and one can lead to the other. A specialist may need to examine both your stride and the biomechanical structure of the lower half of your body. Gait analysis using high-speed video or digital techniques is effective, but can be costly. Talk to your sports medicine physician about what is available in your area. There may be a clinic for runners that can assist you in this endeavor.

At the FIRST running retreats held on the Furman University campus, a gait analysis is performed on each runner. All of the retreat participants receive a CD with a video of their running with accompanying remarks about their running form. In addition, we recommend specific stretches and strength training exercises that address any weaknesses identified in their running.

Q. What about taking nonsteroidal anti-inflammatories to treat/prevent running injuries?

A. Nonsteroidal anti-inflammatories (NSAIDs) are very useful in reducing the inflammation associated with different types of running injuries. Their use is often indicated during the recovery from overuse injuries, but should not be used to permit training by masking the inflammation. You should treat NSAIDs as medicine, not as performance boosters. Doing so may lead to greater injury and other complications.

Q. Do I need orthotics?

A. Orthotics are inserts placed in the shoe to correct certain biomechanical problems, such as overpronation or flat feet. Orthotics may be helpful to a runner with bad alignment who is suffering from pain and repeated injuries. A sports medicine doctor can evaluate whether orthotics will be beneficial.

Q. How does excess body weight affect running injuries?

A. Carrying too much body weight puts significant additional strain on the joints, ligaments, and muscles. At our FIRST running retreats, we find that most runners are disciplined with their training, but they often lack discipline with their food choices and consumption. Two problems result from their poor dietary habits— being malnourished and overweight for optimal training and racing.

THE MOST COMMON RUNNING INJURIES

The American Academy of Physical Medicine and Rehabilitation estimates that 70 percent of runners will become injured. Here are the most common types of injuries we see, a bit about their associated signs and symptoms, and the most common forms of treatment.

Runner's Knee

Runner's knee is a term that refers to several conditions associated with pain around the front of the knee. This pain is often a result of a misalignment that causes irritation to the underside of the kneecap.

Signs and Symptoms: Generally, mild irritation at the joint itself will occur. There may be localized swelling and redness. If left untreated, the inflammation can become painful to the point that any running or walking downhill or climbing stairs results in strong pain in the joint.

Treatment: Since this condition is due to overuse, reducing the current training regimen is usually warranted. The runner doesn't need to stop activity, but he or she may need to substitute other forms of exercise until the inflammation is cured. Any activity that puts strain on the knee will slow healing. Running hills may have to be greatly reduced or eliminated. Low-impact activities such as running on an elliptical trainer, pool running, or swimming can be substituted. Absolute rest may be required in extreme cases, but this is uncommon.

Strengthening the quadriceps (thigh muscles) is an important goal. Hamstring stretching, along with calf muscle stretching, may permit complete straightening of the knee in a normal fashion.

Ice is still one of the best ways to deal with inflammation. After your workout, do a 10-minute cooldown stretch of the lateral thigh, hamstrings, and gastrocnemius. Immediately begin icing the knee. Fill a plastic bag with ice and apply it directly to the patellar area; hold in place with an elastic wrap. Keep the ice on for 20 minutes and follow this routine after every workout.

Iliotibial Band Syndrome

Iliotibial band syndrome (ITBS) is the most common cause for pain located on the side of the knee. Like many running injuries, ITBS takes weeks to reach a level that begins to affect training. Sometimes a runner has had no signs or symptoms, but is struck with lateral knee pain while running on a road with a sloped shoulder.

Overpronation can result in stress on the iliotibial band. Weak thigh muscles, hamstrings, and quadriceps often are related to the risk for ITBS, as are weak gluteal muscles.

Signs and Symptoms: The most common complaint will be a sharp or burning pain on the lateral aspect of the knee. Typically, pain begins after running a certain distance and is likely to worsen as the run continues. Following the run, the pain may disappear but will return during the next training session. As the condition worsens, the pain may become prominent earlier during the run and eventually even during walking, particularly when climbing stairs. Redness and swelling over the lateral aspect of the knee develop occasionally.

Treatment: Rest, ice massage, and nonsteroidal anti-inflammatories can address the acute symptoms. After the pain subsides, the runner should begin stretching the iliotibial band (see Chapter 13). The quadriceps, hamstrings and hip muscles will need strengthening to prevent a recurrence (see Chapter 12 exercises).

In severe cases, a physician might prescribe a steroid injection.

Shin Splints

When the connective tissue, tendons, and ligaments of the lower leg become inflamed, the condition is called shin splints.

Beginning runners are most likely to be affected. Several factors that may lead to shin splints include hard running surfaces, worn-out shoes, uneven running surfaces, flat feet, and excessive hill running. All of these can contribute to microtears in the connective tissue that develop into inflammation because of inadequate recovery from excessive stress.

Signs and Symptoms: The pain of shin splints is seemingly minor initially and not easy to locate, although it is generally in the lower third of the tibia where the muscles attach to the bone. The pain usually arises at the same distance into every run. It may improve or get worse as the run continues. Usually it will disappear several minutes to hours after the run is over. If left untreated, the pain is likely to increase over time and become constant, triggered even by slow walking. If the runner can point to a particular point on the leg where the pain is triggered by touch, he or she may have a stress fracture, which requires medical attention.

Treatment: Since shin splints are primarily an overuse injury, the treatment is similar to that for the other overuse injuries already described—rest from running, ice massage, nonsteroidal anti-inflammatories, and stretching the lower-leg muscles.

Well-conditioned muscle fatigues more slowly; therefore, the more you strengthen the muscles of the legs, the better your chances of avoiding shin splints.

Stress Fractures

The heavy forces on the feet and legs from running make these areas extremely susceptible to microscopic injuries to the bone that do not have time to heal. Eventually the bone begins to fail and small cracks can be seen with x-rays or other images. Increases in mileage, particularly sudden increases, can bring about bone damage that the body can't repair quickly enough, leading to stress fractures. The muscles get fatigued with training, absorb shock more poorly, requiring the bones to bear more of the shock of impact. Harder surfaces, such as concrete, also increase the likelihood of injury. Runners who do not take in enough calcium or have other conditions that might weaken bones are more susceptible to stress fractures. Females are at greater risk of stress fractures than males due in part to their smaller muscle mass and inadequate calcium intake.

Signs and Symptoms: The pain associated with stress fractures is usually more localized than that in shin splints. Tenderness and swelling may be present at the fracture site. Your doctor may use a bone scan, or other diagnostic imaging, to diagnose a stress fracture.

Treatment: Rest may take care of the problem. If the injury is not too serious, typically 4 to 8 weeks without running, during which time you'll have to use cross-training, should be sufficient.

Achilles Tendinitis

Inflammation of the Achilles tendon is primarily due to overuse, complicated by anatomical or biomechanical problems. Muscle inflexibility, overpronation, and weak lower leg muscles can all be factors in Achilles tendinitis. A single extreme stress may also result in injury and pain.

Signs and Symptoms: The sudden appearance of acute tendinitis is defined by the rapid onset of a sharp or burning pain. Squeezing the tendon results in a sharp pain. As the tissue warms up, pain may decrease. It may be possible to rub the tendon between your thumb and index finger and feel a gritty sensation, a sign of inflammation.

Achilles tendinitis is one of the major causes of heel pain. A lump may form in the belly of the tendon or just to the side of where the tendon attaches to the heel bone. Early morning walking may be extremely painful for several steps, but subsides with more walking.

Treatment: Rest is the key to healing Achilles tendon problems. Reduce training volume by 50 percent until the pain is completely gone. Nonsteroidal anti-inflammatories may be taken for 7 to 10 days. Ice massage three to four times a day for 20 minutes is also a great way to reduce the inflammation. When the pain has disappeared, begin increasing your training by 5 to 10 percent each week, until you have returned to your normal volume.

A 1/4-inch-thick heel pad may be placed in the shoe of the injured side. Addition of the heel pad reduces the tension on the Achilles tendon. You may need to keep it in your shoe for several months.

Inspect your shoes for excessive wear. Seek the advice of a person trained in the selection of running shoes based on foot mechanics. Consider the use of orthotics, too.

Achilles tendinitis responds well to conservative stretching (see Chapter 13). If conservative treatment does not improve the pain significantly, then more aggressive forms of therapy may be necessary, even casts and physical therapy. You must be patient. Severe cases of Achilles tendinitis can take many months to resolve.

If treatment for the injury is ignored or you continue to run through the pain, damage to the tendon can weaken the connective tissue so that it is unable to withstand the additional forces of jumping, running, or climbing stairs, making a rupture possible. A ruptured tendon requires surgery and casting for 12 months, followed by several months of physical therapy.

Plantar Fasciitis

One of the most common running injuries is plantar fasciitis. Inflammation occurs where the plantar fascia, a bundle of connective tissue in the sole of the foot, attaches to the heel bone, eventually causing heel pain.

Repeated stresses during footstrike result in plantar fascia strain. This strain is exaggerated by running fast and up hills. Both cause the fascia to stretch. Running on soft sand can inflame the fascia. If the volume of training—in particular, the type of training described above—is too great for the recuperative powers of the tissues, a cycle of plantar fasciitis may begin.

Signs and Symptoms: The universal symptom for plantar fasciitis is a sharp pain in the heel and arch during the first few steps in the morning. The plantar fascia contract during the night's rest, and the first few steps begin the painful process of stretching the plantar fascia. Sitting for long periods during the day may result in the same pain in the arch.

The pain of plantar fasciitis may get better during a warmup for a training session and may remain at a reduced level throughout the session. As the runner begins cooling down, the pain begins to increase and may be quite severe over the next few hours.

Treatment: The first level of treatment is conservative and consists of rest, icing, stretching, heel pads, store-bought orthotics, massage, and nonsteroidal anti-inflammatories. Massage can help to stretch the fascia. Common methods for massaging the bottom of the foot include rolling the foot over a can, round stick, or ball. Early treatment should resolve the inflammation for most runners.

More aggressive levels of treatment might include steroid injections, custom orthotics, night splints, and physical therapy. Steroids can have an immediate positive effect on the pain of plantar fasciitis. However, the pain is likely to return if appropriate follow-up treatment is not maintained. Orthotics may be necessary to control foot motion and support the arch during footstrike and toe-off. Night splints will keep the plantar fascia from contracting overnight.

Chronic Calf Tears

A common injury among runners is chronic calf muscle tears. These tears result in knots in the calf, and scar tissue develops.

Signs and Symptoms: While the knots probably develop over time, they tend to appear suddenly to the runner when a sharp tightness occurs in the calf. This tightness can stop the runner in his tracks. Runners often describe this onset as viselike pressure in the calf.

Treatment: Cross-friction massage must be applied to the knots to stretch the damaged fibers and to relieve the pressure exerted on the muscle. Stretching both the soleus and the gastrocnemius must be done regularly (see Chapter 13). These stretches are recommended before and after running. It is important to begin all workouts with 10 to 15 minutes of easy running, gradually increasing the pace before any intensive running.

REAL RUNNER REPORT

Dear FIRST,

Just wanted to send a big thank you for the detailed marathon training plan from your book. I picked it up after having realized (through three stress fractures) that traditional training plans that simply ramp up mileage do not work for me. At age 36, I was at the end of my rope after suffering my third fracture, this time in my pelvis. After taking almost 6 months off, I finally started back slowly, but knew that I needed to try something completely different.

I found you through a *Runner's World* ad and the rest is history. I had BQ'd the previous spring and decided to go back for more. I used your program and found not only that it eliminated the boredom factor but the speed/tempo work made Heartbreak Hill not so heartbreaking! Being an injury-prone runner, this provided the conditioning I needed without placing extra trauma to my body. In the end, I BQ'd again with a PR of 3:33:57 and will go back next year . . . with your help of course!

Cathy Meier
Pharmacist and Mother
Findlay, Ohio

FOLLOW-UP MESSAGE:

Since I wrote you that email, I have used your program three times (two of them for Boston!) for a NEW PR of 3:26:09. I pretty much point all new and struggling runners to the program and all my mom-runner friends now swear by it as it offers so much flexibility in a training week.

SUMMARY

One of the primary goals of the FIRST program is to promote lifelong running enjoyment. Injury prevention is critical in meeting this goal. Overuse injuries are the major culprit in ending many runners' careers. Therefore, reducing total volume of training by eliminating unnecessary miles prevents injuries.

Our program requires higher-intensity training to permit the runner to reach his or her goals. This training is tailored to the individual's abilities as defined by current performance levels, while allowing for 4 days without running each week. These off-days permit recovery from previous workouts, leaving the runner fresh for the next training run and reducing overuse problems. However, every runner must carefully monitor his or her body, particularly the knees, ankles, and feet, for signs and symptoms of overuse injuries and be prepared to take immediate action to prevent progression of an injury to more severe levels.

REAL RUNNER REPORT

FIRST Team,

I just thought I'd drop a quick email to thank you for your great training program. As an active duty marine pilot, my days are very chaotic, and I seldom ever have a "routine" workday. I easily incorporated your program into my busy schedule, and I enjoyed considerable success while running the 2008 Marine Corps Marathon. I finished with a 3:07, which beat my previous time by over 23 minutes! From mile 20 to the finish I felt relaxed and in complete control of the race unlike my previous attempts in which I felt like I was in "survival" mode. Additionally, 2 days after the marathon I feel great and can resume running again this week, which was not the case in years past.

I'm spreading the good word.

Thanks,

Will Grant
Major, United States Marine Corps

CHAPTER 11

RUNNING NUTRITION

When runners submit their applications for FIRST email coaching or to be a participant at one of our Running Retreats, they are asked to list an area of their running that needs improvement. Most cite a need to improve dietary habits. Before the retreat, participants complete a 3-day food diary. Then we analyze their food consumption and provide detailed information about their macro- and micronutrients, as well as their daily caloric intake. What we observe is that runners, like most Americans, fail to eat a balanced diet that is composed primarily of fruits, vegetables, and grains. We are particularly struck by how many runners rely on energy bars for many of their daily calories.

Runners who train vigorously and assiduously are often not willing to be as disciplined with their eating habits. We are convinced that they fail to reach their potential because they are not properly fueled for their training. We have seen runners in our training studies improve dramatically with improved nutrition as much as with dedicated and smart training.

Most of the runners attending our lectures and participating in our training studies say they are confused about dietary guidelines or have difficulty adhering to them. Unfortunately, the avalanche of books touting unsound dietary schemes has not made it easier for runners to be well informed about proper nutrition.

"Portion Distortion" has made it difficult for Americans to recognize what is a reasonable amount of food to consume. Larger servings, plates, cartons, and bottles have made it a challenge to understand what a normal serving size is. Maintaining an ideal weight is a matter of balancing caloric intake (the food you eat) with caloric expenditure (daily metabolism and calories burned by exercise.) Sorry, there is no magic weight-loss diet. Just as it takes months of dedicated training to prepare for a marathon, that same discipline is necessary for losing weight.

NUTRITION: THE ESSENTIALS

• A well-balanced diet is recommended for all healthy adults; just because you exercise doesn't mean you can eat anything you want.

• A runner's diet should be based primarily on complex (unrefined) carbohydrates, which includes whole grains, fruits, and vegetables.

• Sixty to 70 percent of your calories should come from carbohydrate sources, with only 10 percent from simple carbohydrates.

• Protein should account for 15 percent of total calories, and should be selected from vegetables and lean cuts of meat. Vegetable protein is just as nutritious as animal protein, but has less saturated fat.

• Fat calories should account for 15 to 25 percent of your total caloric intake.

• Trans-fatty acids (common in snack and processed foods) should be avoided due to their significant negative impact on blood cholesterol.

• Healthy eating will meet all of the needs of the runner, with only minimal changes needed prior to competition.

• The diet must provide the energy needed for successful participation in a vigorous training program.

• Once their optimal weight for training has been obtained, runners must fine-tune caloric intake to maintain their desired target weight.

• Not eating enough will make you unable to complete the quality workouts in the FIRST Training Program and may result in loss of lean body weight.

• It is best to eat various foods that provide a variety of nutrients

NUTRITION: Q AND A

Q. Why should I consume so many carbohydrates?

A. Carbohydrates supply the body's immediate energy needs and are the major source for glycogen, which is the storage form of carbohydrates in the body. A high-carbohydrate diet ensures the runner a full glycogen load for training and competition.

Minimizing the consumption of simple sugars will help avoid a roller-coaster effect in blood glucose levels. Choosing fruits for dessert is a healthier option than refined-sugar desserts. Fruits, like other unrefined carbohydrates, add lots of important vitamins and minerals and, in some cases, fiber.

Intense training requires that carbohydrates be replaced daily. Since FIRST training is based on high-quality running, it is important that your daily diet be based predominantly on complex (unrefined) carbohydrates.

Q. What is the glycemic index and should I concern myself with it?

A. The glycemic index is a measure of how a carbohydrate source affects your blood sugar level. Some carbohydrates raise your blood sugar level more than others.

Foods with a high glycemic index release sugar into the bloodstream faster than foods with a lower glycemic index. The quick rise in blood sugar triggers an insulin response. The resulting hyperglycemic condition is associated with long-term weight gain, diabetes, and coronary heart disease. Athletes want to consume meals with a low glycemic index so that energy is released steadily throughout their competition. Also, a low-glycemic-index diet reduces hunger and helps you feel fuller longer, which is valuable for weight management.

In general, refined carbohydrates and simple carbohydrates (sugars) have a higher glycemic index than complex carbohydrates (starches). Unrefined grains such as brown rice and whole-grain breads and cereals tend to have a lower glycemic index than refined carbohydrates. Fruits and vegetables also have a low glycemic index. Other examples of carbohydrates with lower glycemic index values are whole wheat pastas, whole-grain breads, bran cereals, grapes, fresh and dried apricots, apples, grapefruit, oranges, baked beans, lentils, corn, peas, chickpeas, green beans, and low-fat yogurt.

After an intense workout or race, however, you might choose to consume high glycemic foods, for example, a candy bar, pretzels, white bread, baked potato, or sports drink, to get the blood glucose level up quickly so as to assist in replenishing muscle glycogen and aid recovery.

Q. Will consuming more protein increase my running performance?

A. Protein does not provide a significant amount of energy when you run or work out. Protein is the major building material of the body and is essential for tissue growth and repair. A diet based on 15 percent protein will meet both of these needs. The body cannot store protein; any extra is converted into carbohydrates or fat, with little being used for your immediate energy needs.

Q. Is the protein from meat better than proteins from plant sources?

A. Protein is protein regardless of the source. Animal protein has been called high-quality protein because it contains all 20 amino acids needed by humans. Soy is the only plant source that contains all 20 amino acids. Therefore, vegetarians must mix and match their food selections to ensure they receive all 20 amino acids from their diet. For example, a combination of beans and rice, sometimes called complementary protein sources, will supply all of the essential amino acids. For health, more of your protein should be derived from plant sources so as to reduce fat intake. While we are not necessarily advocating a vegetarian diet, we are suggesting that endurance athletes and runners adopt a plant-based diet.

Q. Why are polyunsaturated fats preferred to saturated fats?

A. There are numerous studies linking saturated fat with chronic diseases, especially heart disease. Polyunsaturated fats have been associated with a decrease in the risk for these diseases. By combining unsaturated fats and a low-fat diet, the runner will have an optimal disease-fighting menu. A healthy runner is typically a faster runner.

Q. What are trans-fatty acids (TFAs), and why are they considered so bad?

A. Trans-fatty acids are created by a hydrogenation process of corn or other oils to increase shelf life and meet consumer tastes. Trans-fatty acids are known to reduce the good cholesterol, HDL, while increasing the bad cholesterol, LDL. TFAs have also been shown to damage the blood vessels, increasing the risk of atherosclerosis and heart disease.

Q. How much fluid does the runner need to consume?

A. It is important to stay adequately hydrated. Drink enough during the day to keep your urine clear. Two hours before a workout, drink 16 ounces of your preferred sports drink or water. Two hours is ample time for the fluid to be cleared from the stomach and for the kidneys to remove the excess. Thirst is not a reliable way of determining your hydration needs.

You should consume a quantity of fluid that is equal to your fluid loss from sweating and breathing during exercise. Weighing yourself before and after a run is a good way to determine your sweat loss during exercise. In general, you need to drink 1 pint of fluid for each pound lost during exercise. Sweat rates vary from runner to runner and with weather conditions.

You need to practice drinking during your training, both to train your body to handle fluids during exercise and to learn what is a comfortable amount for you to drink while working out. This is especially important during longer events, when fluid loss from sweating might exceed the ability of your body to process added fluids.

Q. What fluid is best to drink?

A. Well before race day, contact the event promoters to find out what types of fluid replacement are available. During your long runs, practice with the race-day drink to get used to it. If you can't tolerate the event drink, be prepared to drink water or carry your own drink. You do not want to find out on race day that your stomach can't handle the event drink.

Q. Can I drink too much water?

A. Yes, especially during prolonged exercise. For the last several years, runners have heard "hydrate, hydrate, hydrate." Hydration is good and important, but during long runs some runners drink too much fluid. The popularity of the marathon has resulted in the participation of runners with a vast divergence of talent. Marathon times have increased to an average of over 4 hours, with many runners still on the road 5 to 6 hours after the start. Many of these runners have trained with groups that stress the importance of fluid intake throughout the course of the race. Due to the low workload related to their pace, these runners actually gain water weight as a result of consuming more water than what they lose by sweating. This results in lower sodium concentrations in their blood and can lead to hyponatremia. Because the symptoms may resemble those of dehydration, hyponatremia victims are often given liquids, only worsening their condition. Hyponatremia is a life-threatening condition that has been responsible for several marathoners' deaths over the past years. Use your weight loss during exercise as a guide for fluid replacement.

Q. Should I take a mineral/vitamin supplement?

A. In general, a balanced diet will meet the needs of most runners. Due to the stress on the body from high-quality training, taking a multiple vitamin with minerals once a day is fine and has not been shown to pose any health risks as long as "mega" vitamins are avoided. Because you are getting vitamins and minerals from the foods you eat, try to find a vitamin that has no more than 100 percent of the RDA values.

Supplements, unlike drugs, do not have to be shown to be effective by the manufacturer. Consult with your health care provider before taking supplements, especially when combining or substituting them with other medicine.

Q. How many calories do I need to consume daily?

A. The quick answer is "as many as you burn daily." A complete answer is not so easy. Body size and activity level play a significant factor in the determination of daily caloric needs. A simple estimate of daily caloric needs is to multiple your body weight (in pounds) by 11.3. Then add an additional 100 calories for each mile of running.

For example, a 135-pound runner who ran 5 miles would need approximately:

$$135 \times 11.3 = 1{,}525 + 500 \text{ (for 5 miles)} = 2{,}025 \text{ calories}$$

A 61.5-kilogram runner who ran 8 kilometers would need approximately:

$$61.5 \times 2.2 \text{ (conversion to lbs.)} \times 11.3 = 1{,}529 + 500 \text{ (for 8 kilometers)} = 2{,}029 \text{ calories}$$

These are estimates and will require fine-tuning by each individual.

Q. What is an ideal body weight for a runner?

A. The runner should be more concerned about body composition than body weight. For long-distance running, extra body weight puts significant stress on the legs. Extra weight also increases the overall workload on the body, thereby decreasing running economy. For most male runners, a body composition of 8 to 15 percent fat would be an achievable goal, while female runners should aim for a range of 16 to 25 percent body fat.

Q. Do I need special nutrition for competition? How about carbohydrate loading?

A. Exercise increases the energy requirements of the body up to 25 times those of normal expenditure. The body converts all carbohydrates to glucose, which may be used immediately as fuel or stored for later use. Glycogen is the storage form of glucose in the body, mostly in the skeletal muscles and liver. The body has a limited storage capacity for glycogen, which may be rapidly depleted during strenuous exercise.

During exercise that feels easy, over half of the calories used for energy comes from stored body fat. As exercise intensity increases to moderate, the body begins to burn less fat and utilize more glycogen- stored carbohydrates. Long runs tend to deplete glycogen. The term "hitting the wall" is used to describe the effect that glycogen depletion has on a runner.

Once your stored glycogen is depleted, your body shifts back to burning fat. Because converting fat to energy cannot be done as efficiently as using glycogen for energy, your pace decreases.

One aim of training is to increase the pace at which you can run while burning fat. In other words, your easy pace becomes a faster pace. By burning fat rather than glycogen, you put off glycogen depletion longer and put off hitting the wall. Appropriate training increases the pace you can maintain before your crossover from fat burning to carbohydrate burning occurs, helping to save glycogen that will be needed farther down the road.

If you maintain a diet that is high in complex carbohydrates, it is not necessary to carbo-load. As you begin a taper, your activity level will decline; thus you will burn fewer of your carbohydrate stores. Your normal high carbohydrate diet (60 to 70 percent of total calories coming from carbohydrates), combined with a decrease in activity (for your taper), will result in carbo-loading. The day prior to your race should also be high in carbohydrates, but refined carbohydrates may make a better choice because of their reduced fiber content.

The most efficient energy yield from stored glycogen occurs with an even running pace. A fast pace early in the race speeds the depletion of glycogen and leads to hitting the wall.

Q. What should the runner eat prior to competition?

A. Individuals must determine the type and quantity of food to eat before a race, as well as when they will consume the meal. To work out your personal plan, begin with the information below. Through trial and error on long-distance training days, vary the type, quantity, and timing of meals. Maintain an accurate log of these variables and your long run performances to determine your most effective and agreeable prerace meal plan.

For a simple way of estimating your caloric needs on race morning, use this formula:

(hours before race) × (body weight in pounds) = (number of calories to eat)

(hours before race) × (body weight in kilograms × 2.2) = (number of calories to eat)

For example, if you wake up at 6:00 a.m. and your race is at 8:00 a.m., that's 2 hours. So for a 150-pound runner that's 2 × 150 = 300 calories.

Typically, consuming 300 to 500 calories 3 hours before a half-marathon or marathon followed by 100 to 150 calories of sports drink an hour prior to the race should supply adequate prerace fuel.

For shorter races (5K and 10K) lasting less than an hour, fewer, if any, prerace calories are necessary.

Q. Does the runner need to ingest calories during the race?

A. Running a marathon or half-marathon may deplete your glycogen stores, resulting in your hitting the wall. To prevent it, you need to consume carbohydrates during the race, not only to replace glycogen stores in the muscle but also to maintain the level of blood glucose needed by the active muscles. The goal can be met with 6 to 8 ounces of sports drink every 30 to 35 minutes and on warmer days every 20 to 30 minutes. Some runners like to use energy gels during marathons. Consuming an energy gel with water every hour can also help maintain adequate blood glucose levels.

Even though you may have 90 or more minutes of stored carbohydrates, you need to begin taking sports drink early in the race in order to spare your stores of glycogen.

Q. What should the runner consume after a workout or race?

A. Sports drinks are a good option. The body is a carbohydrate sponge immediately after intense and exhausting exercise. Glycogen resynthesis from carbohydrates consumed after exercise takes place most rapidly during the first 30 minutes. Foods with a high glycemic index may speed up the replenishment of glycogen in skeletal muscle due to the rapid rise in glucose and insulin. During the first 2 hours following exercise, try to take in solid foods that are high in carbohydrates, such as bagels, bananas, pudding, etc.

Research indicates that the maximum human carbohydrate synthesis is 225 grams (900 calories) of glucose following exercise. This amount of carbohydrate should be consumed in small portions over the 2-hour window. If you consume too much carbohydrate, the excess is stored as fat.

RUNNING NUTRITION: CONCLUSION

Running, as with all physical activities, requires energy. If there are several ways to meet the energy needs of the body, the question becomes, "What is the best diet?" The shelves of bookstores are filled with volumes, all claiming to offer the "best" diet. This manual is not a sports nutrition manual, nor is there room to explore the biochemistry of nutrition. Only basic nutritional information is provided. For more specific dietary information, FIRST recommends consultation with a sports nutritionist.

REAL RUNNER REPORT

Hi Guys,

Please bear with my novel-length email; I really want to tell you the whole story. I am a 42-year-old male. I've never in my life been medically obese, but nor have I ever been what you'd call "very fit." Like most people, exercise ebbed and flowed in my life. Some years I exercised regularly, other years not so much. As for running, I never even considered entering any kind of competitive event, and never ran for more than 15 to 30 minutes at a time and only on a treadmill.

Things took a turn for the worse for me—healthwise—between March 2007 and November 2009. During those years, my wife and I had two beautiful little girls. We both continued working full-time, and any shred of healthy eating or exercise went completely out the window. We began to rely on eating a lot of take-out food (can you say pizza and Chinese?) and lots of unhealthy "snacks." My poor eating habits, combined with no exercise, resulted in an expanding waistline. Over two years, I put on an extra 30 pounds and went from a 32 to a 36 waist. I knew I wasn't living a healthy lifestyle, but I figured that since I was only 41, I had plenty of time to change my habits and lose weight. Then I got a really, really big wake-up call.

In November 2009 I was in my backyard raking leaves when I felt a sharp pain in my chest followed by tingling in my hands. A short ambulance ride later, I arrived in the ER where doctors performed an angioplasty and put a stent in my right coronary artery to save my life. At the ripe old age of 41, I had suffered a heart attack! Doctors warned me that two other arteries were more than 40 percent clogged, and that if I didn't make drastic changes in my life, things were not going to get better. To be perfectly honest, I got lucky that day. I very easily could have made my wife a widow and left my two little girls (then 2½ and 8 months old) without a dad. Neither of them would have any memories of me as they got older and would have only pictures and stories of their father. The thought of that was absolutely crushing to me and I was released from the hospital with a determination never to let that happen.

I spent December 2009 to March 2010 in "cardiac rehabilitation." Under the watchful eye of RN/personal trainers who monitored my heart on an EKG, I built up a solid base level of fitness. I lost all 30 pounds and began to feel healthier than I'd ever felt in my life. I completed rehab in late March, passed a nuclear stress test with flying colors, and received full medical clearance to "exercise vigorously."

During rehab I really started to develop a love for running. At the end of April, I ran my first 5K (in 26:45) and was absolutely hooked on competitive running. At about that same time, I discovered your book. I had been looking at other running books and training plans but, as you know, most of them wanted me to run 4 or more days a week. And while I love running, I also wanted to have time to bike, swim, and lift weights. Your 3-day-a-week plan was absolutely perfect for me.

(continued on page 154)

In mid-May 2010, I decided that I would use your training plans to train for a fall half-marathon. Over the spring and summer your book and training plans became a part of my life. I began getting up very early on Sunday morning for my long runs. I started out with 9:36 as my target HM pace, but revised the time downward twice over the summer as the workouts began feeling too easy for me (I was also carefully monitoring my HR with a HR monitor and checking in with my doctor, don't worry!).

On race day (for the Parks Half-Marathon, Rockville, Maryland), my target HM pace was 9:01. As you all wisely counsel, I held back at my planned HM pace for the first half of the race as other runners who had also lined up in the 9:00–9:30 queue sped past at blazing speed. In the second half of the race, still feeling very strong, I stepped on the gas and ultimately crossed the finish line in 1:55:52 (8:51 pace; 93/178 in my age group), far faster than I ever imagined I could run that race. Thanks to your phenomenal book and training plans, only 10 months after almost losing my life I had just run my first HM in under 2 hours. My wife and kids were waiting for me at the finish line, and I had never felt so good in my life.

I carry your book with me just about everywhere I go, reading and rereading various chapters from time to time and picking up on things I may have missed on earlier readings. In short, your book and training plans are now part of my life. I plan to run another half-marathon in the spring and then may consider a full marathon for next fall (with almost 2 solid years of running under my belt).

I'm sorry for the length of this email, but I really wanted to tell you the whole story and enthusiastically thank you for your excellent book. Thank you for playing a part in helping me turn my life around. I do hope to thank you all in person at a future Furman Institute running retreat. Until then, I eagerly await any future publications from you all.

Rod Vieira
Environmental Attorney for the National Oceanic and Atmospheric
Administration
Chevy Chase, Maryland

SECTION IV
Supplemental Training

CHAPTER 12

STRENGTH TRAINING
FOR RUNNERS

Nowhere is the adage "Use it or lose it" more relevant than with muscles. Running tends to employ one set of muscles over and over while neglecting others. Runners must also combat the loss of muscle mass that is a natural part of the aging process. It is imperative that we do strength exercises as we age to diminish the loss of muscle tissue.

For your overall fitness and good health, you should exercise the major muscle groups in the back, chest, shoulders, arms, torso, and legs. For the enhancement of your running, we have provided strength training exercises that can be performed in a relatively short period of time and will contribute to better running and injury prevention.

Runners attending our retreats are surprised by how difficult it is for them to perform some of our strength exercises. That's because they have neglected to do functional strength training—exercises specific to the movements of their sport. It is as important to train the neuromuscular component of the movement as it is the individual muscles. Exercises that isolate muscles and don't mimic the movement of the activity result in less functional improvement. For example, squats will have a greater transfer effect on improving an individual's ability to run than knee extensions. As Scott Murr often points out to runners, running is done one leg at a time. For that reason, one-legged squats will have an even greater transfer effect on your running than two-legged squats. We have selected exercises that are specific to running movements.

I like feeling stronger not only for sports but also for everyday activities. Two or three times per week for about 20 to 30 minutes, I do a circuit of exercises that works the large muscle groups. Typically these strength training sessions are not on key run days. Training partner and coauthor Scott Murr likes to do his strength training on the same days he runs. I recommend establishing a strength training routine that fits your weekly schedule. Consistency is the key.

Strength Training: The Essentials

• Strengthening the core muscles is important for maintaining good running form.

• Strengthening muscles that stabilize the hips and knees is very important for injury prevention.

• Muscular imbalances are often associated with running-specific injuries.

• Strengthening a weak muscle can eliminate imbalances between opposing muscle groups.

• Many runners avoid or neglect strength training.

Strength Training: Q and A

Q. Why should a runner strength train?

A. When you become fatigued, your form deteriorates (poor running economy). The deterioration comes not only from tired legs, but also from tired arms, a tired back, and tired abdominal muscles. Having a strong torso helps hold your form together in the later stages of a workout or a race. Strength training improves running economy (one of the key determinants of running performance), permitting faster running over the same distance with less consumption of oxygen. Improved running economy means you can run for a longer time before exhaustion sets in.

Q. What are the potential liabilities associated with weight training? What should a runner avoid in his or her weight training program?

A. Liabilities include injury due to poor form and additional bulk (muscle and weight gain) following an unnecessarily extensive weight training program.

Our advice is to train the muscle groups that will be of greatest benefit in running. If you follow a body builder's weight training routine, you will probably find minimal if any improvement in your running performance. In fact, it is possible that a standard weight training routine would result in diminished running performances.

Q. What exercises should be included in strength training for runners?

A. There is no single method of strength training that has been shown to be unequivocally superior for runners. Many of our recommended exercises are core exercise and multi-joint exercises (those which use many body parts). Core exercises and multi-joint exercises tend to be more specific to normal body movement. With the FIRST strength training exercises, you won't isolate a single muscle group, the typical approach of many weight training routines.

The American College of Sports Medicine recommends 8 to 10 exercises that work the major muscle groups. While we endorse the ACSM position statement, we have selected 11 key strength training exercises that will enhance running performance. These strength training recommendations are designed so that a runner can do them in a timely manner with minimal equipment.

Q. Do I really need to do lower-body strength exercises?

A. Many runners think, "I don't need to work my legs because I use them all the time running." During running, your legs are being worked, but primarily they are being trained solely for endurance, not strength. Strength training will help improve your leg strength, so that you can generate more force with each stride. Strength training will also help balance the muscular fitness of all of the major muscles of the lower body.

Q. In what order should I do my exercises?

A. Typically, you should train the larger and stronger muscle groups first and then the smaller muscle groups. Why? Your smaller muscles act as supporting muscles when you train the larger muscle groups. If you fatigue the smaller muscle groups first, they won't help much as you stress the larger muscle groups. This puts you at an increased risk for injury. We have listed our strength training exercises in the order we think they should be performed.

Q. How should I breathe when doing strength training exercises?

A. Avoid the temptation to hold your breath when strength training. Even veteran athletes fail to breathe when exerting effort and are often unaware of it. You should breathe continuously and should exhale on the exertion or lifting movement and inhale on the return or lowering movement.

Q. Should I strength train year-round?

A. Varying your routine periodically is important to stimulate adaptation. FIRST believes that year-round strength training is fine as long as you reduce your strength training program the final 2 weeks before a key race.

For each of the following key strength training exercises, we recommend doing 10 to 15 repetitions.

KEY STRENGTH TRAINING EXERCISES

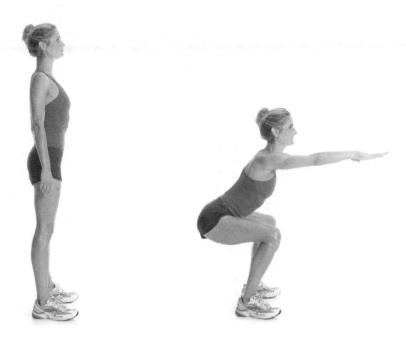

SQUAT
WORKS GLUTES AND QUADRICEPS

Stand with your feet shoulder-width apart.

Keeping your feet flat on the floor, your back straight, and your abdominals tight, squat until your thighs are parallel to the floor.

Keep your weight on your heels rather than your toes. Do not allow your knees to move beyond the point of your toes. Your knees should point in the same direction as your feet throughout the exercise.

Your hands can be placed on your hips or you can hold your arms out in front to help maintain balance.

Return to starting position.

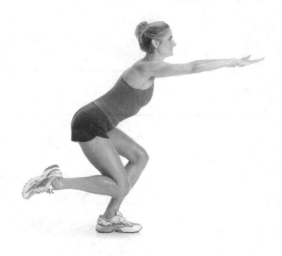

SINGLE LEG SQUAT
WORKS GLUTES, QUADRICEPS, HIP EXTERNAL ROTATORS, HIP ABDUCTORS (ADVANCED)

Stand upright with feet shoulder-width apart.

Bend your right knee lifting your calf up until your shin is parallel to the floor.

Keeping your left foot flat on the floor, your back straight and your head upright, squat down as far as you can while maintaining balance.

Straighten your left leg and return to the starting position.

Keep your abdominals tight throughout the entire exercise.

Do not allow knee or hip to collapse toward the midline of your body.

Repeat with the left leg, then continue with the right leg.

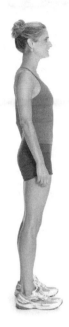
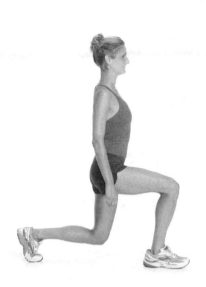

LUNGES
WORKS HAMSTRINGS, QUADRICEPS, GLUTES

Stand with your feet shoulder-width apart.

Step forward with your right leg and lower your body until your right thigh is parallel to the floor and your left knee is almost touching the floor.

The hip, knee, and ankle of your right leg should form a 90-degree angle in the down or forward position. Avoid stepping so far forward that your front knee extends beyond your toes.

The forward knee should point in the same direction as the forward foot throughout the exercise.

Be sure to keep your body upright and your abdominals tight during the lunge.

Return to the starting position by driving your weight back up with your right leg.

Repeat with your left leg.

You have now done 1 rep.

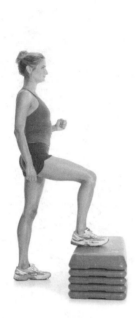
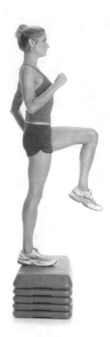

Box Step-Ups
WORKS GLUTES, QUADRICEPS, HAMSTRINGS

Find a box that is 8 to 18 inches high.

Place your right foot entirely up on top of the box with your arms in a running position.

With your weight focused on your right heel, rather than your forefoot, use your right leg to lift yourself to an upright position on the box. Your right knee should point in the same direction as your right foot throughout the exercise.

This exercise is most effective when you lift from the upper leg and avoid pushing up with the foot on the ground.

As you step up, raise your left thigh up to waist height.

Your arms should switch position as you raise yourself up.

Using your right leg to lower yourself back to the ground, step down with your left leg and return to the starting position. Place your right foot on the floor.

Keep your torso upright during this exercise. Repeat with your left leg up on the box.

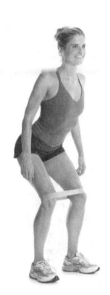 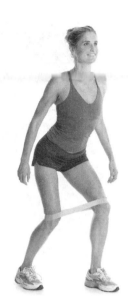

MONSTER (SUMO WRESTLER) WALK
WORKS HIP EXTERNAL ROTATORS, HIP ABDUCTORS

Place a mini-band around your knees or lower legs to make the exercise more challenging.

Stand with your feet slightly more than shoulder-width apart.

Keeping your abdominals tight, bend at the hips and lower your torso so you are standing in a half-squat stance.

Maintaining your wide stance, step forward with your left leg, then with your right leg.

Repeat the exercise stepping backward.

As you move forward and backward, keep a wide stance.

You can place your hands on your waist or out in front of you.

Make sure that you do not allow your knees to turn in (or collapse inwards) during this exercise.

Keep knees bent through the entire exercise.

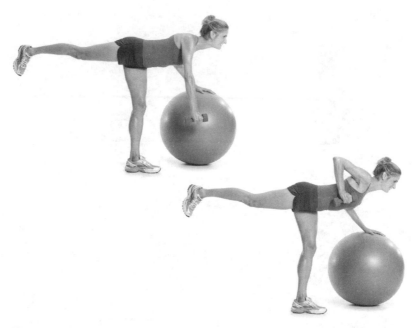

ONE-ARM, ONE-LEG BENT-OVER ROW
WORKS TRICEPS, SHOULDERS, BACK

Start by standing upright and hold a dumbbell in your right hand, keeping your right elbow close to your side.

Stand on your left leg and bend at the waist to approximately a 90-degree angle. Stabilize your upper body with your left hand on a stability ball.

Bend your left knee slightly to reduce pressure on your back. Then lift your right leg to create a "T" with your body.

Pull the dumbbell up toward your shoulder; your elbow will come up just beyond your back. Initiate the row with your shoulder rather than with your arm.

Keep your shoulders and back parallel to floor; avoid rotating at the hips as you lift the weight up.

Slowly extend (straighten) your arm and lower the dumbbell toward the floor.

Be sure to keep your back straight throughout this exercise.

Do the exercise with your right arm, then switch to your left arm and repeat.

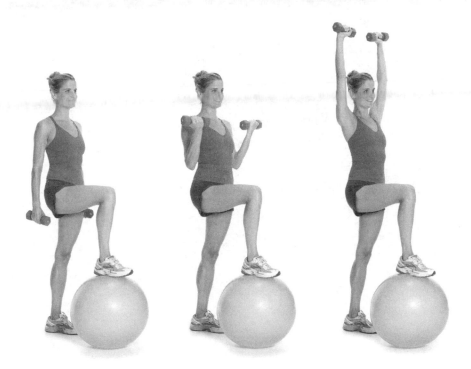

CURL TO PRESS
WORKS BICEPS, SHOULDERS

Stand with your feet about shoulder-width apart behind a stability ball and with your abdominals tight as you hold a pair of dumbbells by your side.

Turn your hands so that your palms face each other.

Prop your right foot up on the stability ball.

Curl the dumbbells toward your shoulders performing the bicep curl with both arms at the same time.

Continue the motion and lift and press the dumbbells overhead, extending your arms straight up toward the ceiling.

Slowly lower your elbows to your sides, then lower the dumbbells to the starting position.

After half of your reps are completed, put the other leg on the stability ball.

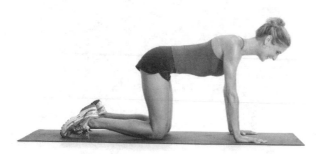

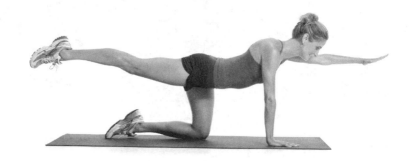

BIRD DOG
WORKS CORE, HAMSTRINGS, SHOULDERS

Begin on your hands and knees on all fours. Your hands should be directly below your shoulders; hold your head in line with your back.

Tighten your abdominal muscles.

Simultaneously, raise your right leg straight out behind you and lift your left arm out in front of you (each is outstretched horizontally).

Hold this raised position for 3 seconds before slowly returning to starting position.

Repeat with your left leg and right arm.

You have completed 1 rep.

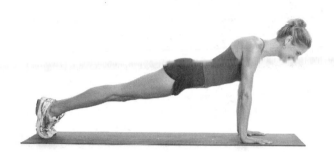

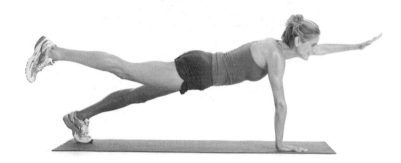

ADVANCED BIRD DOG
WORKS CORE, HAMSTRINGS, SHOULDERS

Begin in a push-up position (on toes) with arms/elbows at full extension (the "up" position of a push-up).

Tighten your abdominal muscles.

Simultaneously lift your left arm and right leg from the floor to a horizontal position.

Maintain full extension for 3 seconds before slowly returning to starting position.

Repeat with your left leg and right arm.

Make sure your avoid bending at the hips: try to keep your back straight the entire exercise.

Alternate arms and legs.

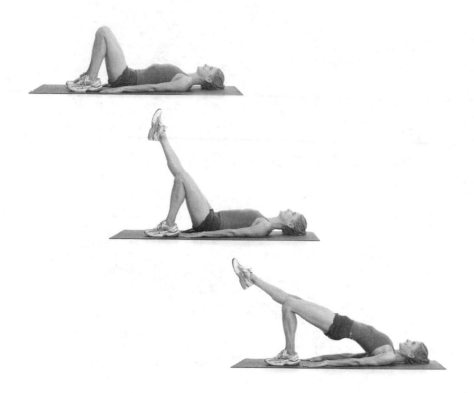

SINGLE-LEG BRIDGES
WORKS GLUTES, CORE

Lie on the floor on your back with your knees bent, feet flat on the floor and arms at your sides.

Straighten your right leg and hold it so that your knees are at the same height.

Keeping your left foot flat on the ground, raise your hips up off the ground to create a straight line from your knees to shoulders. Keep your right leg extended straight out.

Keep abdominals engaged to support the lower back.

Hold for 3 seconds.

Slowly lower yourself and return to the starting position.

Repeat with the other leg.

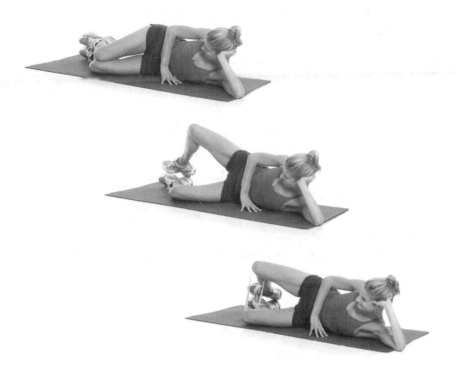

CLAMSHELL
WORKS ABDUCTORS

Lie on your side with your knees and ankles together, your hips bent at a 45-degree angle and your knees bent at a 90-degree angle. Your heels should be in line with your butt.

Raise your top knee toward the ceiling as high as you can (top knee moves away from the bottom knee) and then return to the starting position.

Keep your feet together and avoid rotating your pelvis or back; do not allow your hips to roll back (make sure that your top hip stays facing the ceiling); keep your spine straight.

Hold for one breath, then slowly lower your knee to the starting position.

Place a mini-band around your knees to make the exercise more challenging.

Repeat on both sides.

STRENGTH TRAINING: THE SCIENCE

Most adults lose about half a percent of their muscle mass each year after the age of 25. This loss accelerates after the age of 60. Muscle mass is associated with metabolism. Muscle burns calories at a higher rate than fat. Strength training builds muscle and improves metabolism—a key to maintaining your desired weight.

Studies have shown that as few as 6 weeks of proper strength training can significantly reduce or completely relieve kneecap pain or "runner's knee." Strength training also reduces the recurrence of many other common injuries, including hip and lower back pain (prehab for injury prevention). By strengthening muscle, as well as bone and connective tissue (ligaments attach bone to bone; tendons attach muscle to bone), strength training not only helps to prevent injury but also helps to reduce the severity of injury when it does occur. Running injuries are a runner's worst nightmare!

In addition to injury prevention, strength training improves performance. Studies show that with as little as 10 weeks of strength training, 10K times decrease by an average of 2 to 3 percent. Research has also shown that running economy will be improved as a result of strength training.

REAL RUNNER REPORT

Hi,

Just want to let you know that I bought *Run Less, Run Faster* and followed the program for yesterday's NYC Marathon (my fifth in NYC, sixth overall). I was intent on qualifying for Boston this year—turned 40 in March and my PR was 3:56:22, more than 5 minutes over the 3:50:59 that I needed to qualify. I am THRILLED to report that I got to the start line injury-free (first time I can remember doing that) and easily qualified with a time of 3:48:34, knocking almost 8 minutes off of my PR. I attribute my success to your great, great plan. So I'll be using it again for my next big race on Patriots' Day . . .

Thank you!

Stacey Skole
New York, New York

FOLLOW-UP MESSAGE:

Hi Bill and Scott,

Just an update—I ran my first Boston Marathon yesterday, after having used your FIRST program to qualify in NYC in November 2009. I used FIRST again to train for Boston—and had another PR, despite the fact that I had to re-tie my shoe at mile 24! Finished in 3:47:52, beating my NYC time by over 40 seconds, and paced myself on my own (I ran with a pace team in NYC), so I'm really, really thrilled. I told a new friend about your phenomenal program as well—so I'm sure you'll have a new convert soon.

Thanks again for everything!

CHAPTER 13

FLEXIBILITY AND FORM

Who stretches? Two kinds of runners: (1) those with injuries who've been given specific stretches from a therapist or (2) those who are naturally flexible and for whom stretching is relaxing and easy. Runners who aren't flexible tend to avoid stretching because it isn't comfortable or easy. And we're the ones who need it most.

Several years ago, after incurring injuries that were serious enough to prevent me from running, I learned from a physical therapist that my ankles have tightly spaced bones and connective tissue that hinder flexibility. The leg is a kinetic chain and tightness in one joint will cause unnatural forces on other muscles and joints. Running form is directly influenced by range of motion (flexibility).

It was only by doing a stretching regimen directed by a physical therapist that I could return to running. If I don't stretch my lower calves and work on my ankle flexibility, I get knots in my calves. If I don't stretch my hip flexors, I develop hamstring problems because the muscles improperly bear stress that should be put on the gluteal muscles.

Maybe scientific studies do not definitively confirm that stretching helps prevent injuries; however, the first test a physical therapist or chiropractor gives an injured runner is an assessment of flexibility. Similarly, the first step in rehabilitation is stretching. Just as with strength training, we recommend stretching as prehab, rather than rehab.

Still, there is much disagreement about the value of stretching. Part of the reason is because it's difficult to design research to determine the effects of stretching. Relying on survey data about stretching is questionable.

Those who have been injured will begin stretching to cure a problem. Those who have never been injured see no reason to begin stretching. If you survey runners, the results will show that those who stretch have injuries and those who don't stretch are injury free. You can see how this leads to a false conclusion.

Maybe there is no strong data to support a specific recommendation, but it's well recognized by sport scientists and athletes that flexibility is important for athletic performance. In particular for runners, flexibility of the ankles, hamstrings, and hip flexors affects form and performance. A lack of flexibility often leads to strained muscles or connective tissue. Proper form also improves efficiency and thus economy. And it helps runners avoid injuries.

Good form requires practice and good flexibility. Many factors influence a joint's flexibility and people vary greatly in their flexibility. You should not try to compete with your training partner when it comes to flexibility or stretching. Runners need to monitor their form to make sure that they stay relaxed and aren't losing efficiency due to needless muscular tension. Fatigue often causes runners to tighten their upper bodies, which reduces efficiency. Going through a mental checklist periodically while training and racing can help remind you that the hands, arms, neck, etc., need to be relaxed. In particular, runners tend to lean forward and push their hips back when fatigued, a body position not conducive to economical and effective running.

We recommend that runners take time to incorporate **two key drills and nine key stretches** into their training. These drills and stretches can be completed in a short amount of time, but will pay big dividends. The drills can be combined with your warmup stride running. In keeping with our approach of developing a program that is realistic and also effective, we have not provided a comprehensive set of stretches or drills. Our experience is that most runners don't have the time to devote to extensive stretching and drilling, as do collegiate teams and elite runners. Those runners often devote several hours per day to training. We strive to assist runners with limited time to attain optimal results. Incorporating the two drills and nine stretches along with strides does not take much time, but the benefits are considerable.

FLEXIBILITY: THE ESSENTIALS

- Most runners stretch after they have become injured.

- Inflexible runners don't like to stretch because it is difficult for them.

- Definitive studies show the benefits of stretching for injury prevention or performance enhancement.

- Most runners dovolop tight hamstring and calf muscles, stretching can improve flexibility.

- Tight hamstring and calf muscles can reduce stride length.

- Stretching can reduce muscular stiffness.

- Flexibility improves only after weeks or months of regular and consistent stretching.

- Stretches should begin slowly and held for approximately 30 seconds.

Good Running Form

- Keep your trunk erect.
- Keep your head level.
- Keep your upper body relaxed.
- Keep your hips tall.
- Keep arms and fists relaxed.
- Keep elbow angles from 60 to 140 degrees.
- Imitate leg action with your arms.
- Don't let your arms cross the midline of your body.
- Use your arms for balance.
- Move your legs forward, not up and down.
- Avoid exaggerated knee lift.
- Flex knee of recovery leg so shin is parallel to ground.
- Try to be quick and light on your foot.
- Don't overstride. Your leading foot should not land too far beyond your center of gravity.

FLEXIBILITY AND FORM: Q AND A

Q. What is flexibility and what are the benefits associated with it?

A. Flexibility is typically defined as the ability of a joint to move freely through its full range of motion. Flexibility is joint-specific and is not a general trait. What a cyclist needs to do for flexibility may be very different from what a runner needs to do. Stretching for flexibility:

- improves range of motion
- may improve performance
- may decrease the risk of musculo-skeletal injury
- may decrease muscular tension (stretching does not reduce soreness)
- may improve body alignment
- may help stabilize joints
- can promote relaxation

Q. What are the potential problems associated with limited flexibility?

A. You are only as strong as your weakest link; limited flexibility may have a detrimental impact on one's running. Some running-related problems associated with limited flexibility include lower back dysfunction, postural problems, shortened stride, and muscular strains (e.g., a pulled hamstring).

Q. How can flexibility be improved?

A. To improve the flexibility of a joint, several fitness principles come into play; in particular, muscle elongation is required (overload principle). In other words, muscles must be stretched beyond their normal range of motion. Several methods help accomplish this. See key drills and key stretches later in this chapter.

Q. When should one stretch?

A. For flexibility and running preparation, follow this sequence:

- Warm up with 10 to 20 minutes of easy jogging
- Perform two key drills
- Perform key workout
- Do a cooldown recovery run
- Perform key stretches after the workout

Q. Should I run barefoot?

A. There aren't many people who are willing to run barefoot because of the foot's exposure to rocks, glass, nails, etc., that will result in cuts, abrasions, and bruises. Popular interest in the barefoot concept led shoe manufacturers to develop and promote minimalist shoes that mimic running barefoot. Those recommending a switch from a cushioned shoe to a minimalist shoe claim that cushioning leads runners to heel strike, which increases stress at the knee joint, the most common site for running injuries.

Even though there are claims that barefoot running reduces injuries and that cushioned shoes cause injuries, there are no studies to verify those claims. Good running form, as described in this chapter, will help to reduce the likelihood of injury, regardless of the shoes you wear.

The real issue is whether runners should be rearfoot or midfoot strikers. Rearfoot strikers have increased demand on the knee, especially if their heel strikes the ground in front of the knee. Midfoot strikers put more pressure on the calf muscles and Achilles tendon. The choice between cushioned shoes and minimalist shoes or rearfoot strike and midfoot strike is dependent on the runner's anatomical structures as well as the runner's form.

If you choose to transition from cushioned shoes to minimalist shoes, you should do so gradually. Start with 5 minutes once or twice a week wearing the minimalist shoe and gradually add an additional 5 minutes to your training sessions in subsequent weeks. This transition could interrupt your training until you have successfully made the switch.

TWO KEY DRILLS TO IMPROVE YOUR RUNNING FORM

Dynamic mobility exercises raise the body temperature, increase blood flow to the muscles, activate the nervous system, and prepare you for running.

Perform two **key drills,** dynamic mobility exercises, after a brief 10- to 20-minute warmup and prior to the planned workout.

Strides are great drills. They are runs of 80 to 100 meters, fast but relaxed. You should accelerate gradually over the first three-fourths of the distance and then decelerate to the end. Use strides to practice good form and relaxed running. Strides work fast-twitch fibers in a nonstressful way.

Recover completely between repetitions. Twenty seconds is usually enough recovery time for 100 meters. Strides, which should be done on a grass field or flat area, can be included as part of a warmup or after an easy-day run. Strides will help rejuvenate your legs, which may feel sluggish from slow running.

Running drills emphasize good form. They also help strengthen the muscles needed for strong, efficient running. The hips and ankles are exercised through a greater range of motion more so during drills than during normal runs. While there are many running drills, we've included two to be used during your strides. Doing strides with butt kicks and high knees can enhance your running form.

BUTT KICKS

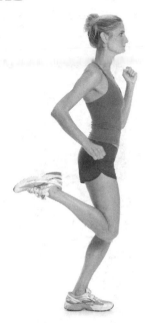

Primarily a hamstring drill, butt kicks involve trying to kick your own butt with each step. Lean slightly forward, take short steps, and kick your heels back and up as high as you can.

Butt kicks improve leg turnover and heel recovery. Heel recovery is the part of the running motion where your leg rises up and coils for the next forward stride. Since one aim of this drill is to increase leg turnover, not stride length, your steps should be quick. Focus on a smooth but quick action.

Perform butt kicks for 20 meters, then gradually stride/accelerate for 60 meters before decelerating for the last 20 meters of the stride.

HIGH KNEES

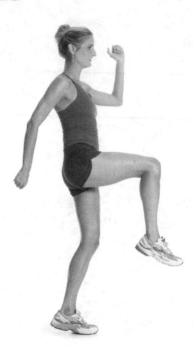

The aim of high knees is to increase leg turnover and improve your knee lift. This drill strengthens the calves and hip flexors, and emphasizes proper running posture and the lift-off phase of running.

High knees involves taking short steps and lifting your knees up as high as they can go. Think of yourself as "prancing." The idea is to stay "tall" while rapidly lifting and driving down the knees. You should be bringing your legs up in front of you and maintaining a nice upright posture.

Turnover is rapid so you take as many steps as possible over 20 meters. The aim is not to move forward quickly but to take quick steps while lifting your knees high. Like butt kicks, this drill is about leg turnover, not stride length.

You will feel this one in the front of your hips and thighs (hip flexors), as they will be working hard to lift your legs up high in front of you.

Perform this drill for 20 meters and then gradually stride/accelerate for 60 meters before decelerating for the last 20 meters of the stride.

NINE KEY STRETCHES TO ENHANCE FLEXIBILITY FOR RUNNING

After a workout (run or cross-training) and cooldown, static stretching is recommended. Do the **key stretches** after the workout or later that day.

KEY STRETCH 1: STANDING CALF

Stand on the top of a step or curb.

Slide your right foot back so that the ball of your foot remains on the step.

Keep your right knee straight, shift your body weight to your right leg, and drop your right heel toward the ground.

Keep your upper body upright. Use a handrail or wall to help maintain your balance.

Keep your right knee straight to maximize the stretch of your calf.

Hold the stretch for 30 seconds.

Now, bend the right knee to feel a stretch in the back of your calf and Achilles tendon.

Hold the stretch for 30 seconds.

Repeat with your left leg.

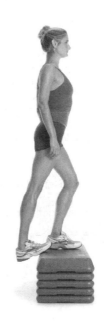

KEY STRETCH 2: QUADRICEPS/HIP FLEXOR

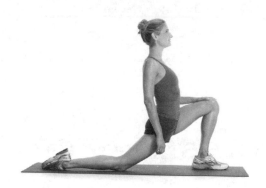

Step forward with your left foot into a runner's lunge.

Drop your right knee to the floor.

Keep your trunk upright, your shoulders back, and press your hips forward.

Your feet should be far enough apart to keep your left knee from extending beyond the toes of your left foot.

Hold this stretch for 30 seconds.

Repeat with your right leg forward.

KEY STRETCH 3: LYING HAMSTRING

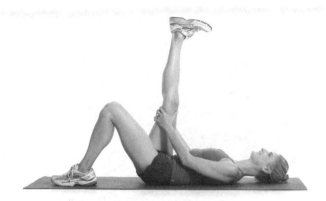

Lie on the floor on your back with your left knee bent and right leg straight.

Place a strap around your right foot or place your hands behind your right thigh near your knee.

Lift your right leg toward the ceiling, keeping your leg straight.

Pull your right leg toward your chest while keeping your right leg straight.

Hold for 30 seconds.

Repeat with your left leg.

Do this stretch twice a day.

KEY STRETCH 4: GLUTES/PIRIFORMIS

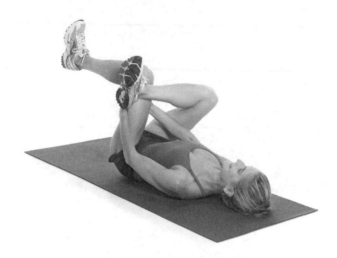

Lie on the floor on your back with your knees bent and feet on the floor.

Cross your right ankle over your left knee.

Clasp your hands behind your left leg and pull slowly toward your chest. You may feel the stretch in your right hip.

If you are unable to reach or grab your thigh, lasso a towel or strap around your thigh and slowly pull the towel or strap toward your chest.

Hold the stretch for 30 seconds.

Repeat with your left ankle crossed in front of your right knee.

Do this stretch twice a day.

KEY STRETCH 5: HIP FLEXORS

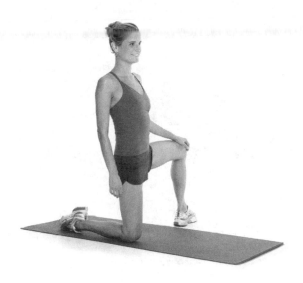

Step forward with your left foot into a runner's lunge.

Drop your right knee to the floor.

Now rotate your left leg 90 degrees to the left to open your hips.

Keep your trunk upright, your shoulders back, and press your hips forward.

Hold this stretch for 30 seconds.

Repeat with your right leg forward.

KEY STRETCH 6: ILIOTIBIAL BAND (ITB) (FOAM ROLLER)

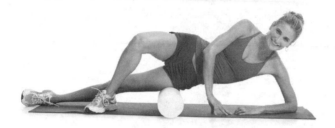

Lie on your left side, use your left forearm and elbow to support your upper body.

Place your right foot on the floor in front of your left knee.

Place a foam roller under your left hip and roll your body over the foam roller along your outer thigh (between your hip and your knee).

Roll back up so that the foam roller comes back toward your left hip.

You can increase the resistance by stacking your right leg on top of your left leg.

Roll back and forth for 30 seconds.

Repeat on your left side.

KEY STRETCH 7: SPINAL ROTATION

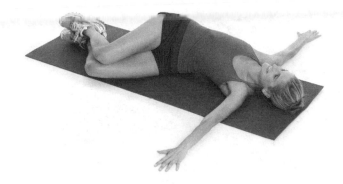

Lie on the floor on your back with your knees bent.

Extend your arms out at shoulder level.

Keeping your knees together, drop your knees to your left side.

Hold this position for 30 seconds.

Bring your knees back up to the starting position.

Drop your knees together to your right side.

Hold for 30 seconds.

Do this stretch twice a day.

KEY STRETCH 8: LOW BACK

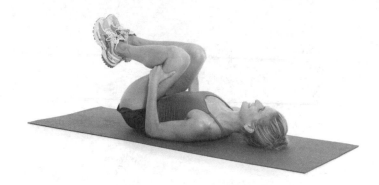

Lie on the floor on your back with your knees bent.

Bring your knees toward your chest.

Place your hands behind your thighs to hold your knees close to your chest.

Hold for 30 seconds.

Do this stretch twice a day.

KEY STRETCH 9: HIP ABDUCTION/ILIOTIBIAL BAND (ITB)

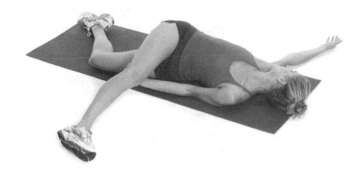

Lie on the floor on your back with your knees bent.

Extend your arms out at shoulder level and look toward your right hand.

Keeping your knees together, drop your knees to your left side.

Extend your right leg so that your straight leg is perpendicular to your torso. Place your left hand under your right leg for support.

Hold this position for 30 seconds.

Bring your knees back up to the starting position.

Extend your arms out at shoulder level and look toward your left hand.

Keeping your knees together, drop your knees to your right side.

Extend your left leg so that your straight leg is perpendicular to your torso. Place your right hand under your left leg for support.

Hold this position for 30 seconds.

Do this stretch twice a day.

REAL RUNNER REPORT

Dear FIRST,

I am a 50-year-old male, veteran marathon runner (98 marathons) who wants to be more efficient and extend my marathoning career. I had been on my own program, designed by me, based a lot on what you have done in your FIRST program. My own schedule of 3 days a week with long runs, speedwork (I did only mile repeats), and tempo runs served me well for many years. However, your FIRST program zeroed in on what my program was missing: active rest via cross-training.

I first used your program to train for the 2009 Boston Marathon. I trained for a 3:30 and ran 3:25. I ran 2 minutes faster on FIRST than the previous year, but it was also my fastest Boston in the previous five Bostons. This is significant because I am 5 years older now.

My second time trying FIRST was for the 2009 Twin Cities Marathon. There I ran my fastest marathon since 2001. Again, now 8 years older, and faster. I used the 3:30 program (doing most of the speedwork faster) and ran a 3:22.

I can't say enough about how much I appreciate your efforts in designing this program! I will be starting up my third FIRST program training schedule on March 1, 2010, as I prepare for my 100th marathon at Grandma's in June. I have told several friends about your book and have made believers out of most of them. My friend Dan, after 20 years of doing it his way, training hard, but never qualifying, he ran FIRST and now we're headed out to Boston in April.

Thank you very much!!

Sincerely,

Mark Johnsrud
Field Operations Sergeant
Wisconsin Department of Corrections
Richland Center, Wisconsin

FOLLOW-UP MESSAGE:

Last Saturday I ran Grandma's Marathon, my 100th marathon overall, starting on a 63-degree morning with 81 percent humidity, party cloudy skies and about a 14 mph headwind. I went out a little fast, but it felt good. I finally settled in and just put it on cruise control and raced like I trained, feeling very comfortable and well trained. I believe the confidence during the program gave my racing a boost because I just felt good. Regardless, I crossed the finish line in 3:19:32, proving you right once again! Thank you, thank you, thank you!!!

FLEXIBILITY AND FORM: FINAL COMMENTS

Stretching is important for healthy flexibility and should not be overlooked. But be aware that poor technique can result in ineffective stretching. It's important to have someone with a trained eye correct your inefficient and potentially injurious form. Find a running coach who will either watch or videotape your running and stretching. You must practice good form just as you practice running faster and farther. There are hundreds of movements that can improve flexibility. A flexibility program should include exercises and movements that work all the major joints of the body. A comprehensive review of the physiology and biomechanics associated with stretching is beyond the scope of this book.

SECTION V
Boston and Beyond

CHAPTER 14

TRIATHLONS, TRAILS, AND ULTRAS

Running is usually the gateway sport to participation in triathlons and trail and ultra races. That's to be expected since running is the most popular of the individual endurance sports. FIRST has received countless requests for training advice from runners who wish to venture into new endurance competitions. Runners want to know if we have created a FIRST counterpart training program for multisport activities and longer-than-marathon running competitions.

We haven't, primarily because we haven't conducted research in these sports and wouldn't have proof for what we would be recommending. However, because of the many requests, we are providing a chapter with advice for runners who wish to branch out to these other sports.

We have extensive triathlon experience but little and no experience with trail and ultra running. For advice on those two sports, we reached out to our good friend Hal Koerner, two-time winner of Western States 100 and a national champion at 50 miles. Hal owns and manages Rogue Valley Runners, an independent running store in Ashland, Oregon. Hal has run over 100 ultramarathons and finished in the top three in 75 percent of them. Hal is familiar with the FIRST training program and answered our questions about how to advise FIRST runners who want to race on trails and go beyond the 26.2-mile distance.

TRAILS AND ULTRAS

Preparing to run a 50K (31.06 miles) race does not require much alteration to the FIRST marathon training program. Adding a little extra distance (3 to 5 miles, 5 to 8 kilometers) to a few of the 20-mile (32K) training runs will prepare you for running an additional 5 miles beyond the traditional marathon distance.

Moving up in distance from a 50K to a 50-miler is significant. When we asked Hal if the FIRST program was appropriate for the 50-mile race, he said simply to add a fourth run per week. He advocates back-to-back weekend long runs. You may begin with adding a 10-mile run on Sunday after having completed the FIRST marathon key run #3 on Saturday. The combination of weekend runs would initially include a 15-mile run followed the next day with a 10-mile run. Through the 16-week training this progression would gradually increase from 15 + 10 to 15 + 15 to 20 + 10 to 20 + 15 to 20 + 20 to perhaps 25 + 20. Hal suggested that 30 miles was the maximum that he would recommend for a training run. Even for his 100-mile races, his longest training run is 30 miles. But he also enters 50-mile races to prepare for 100-mile races.

While the additional mileage of ultras is a challenge, the greater challenge is that almost all ultras are run on trails. Trail running requires strength. The running pace is much slower, making the overall time of running considerably greater. Trails typically require a lot of running up and down—long climbs and downhills. This type of running requires practice. You cannot rely on pace for determining intensity, because the terrain—depending on elevation change and the condition of the trail—influences how fast you can run. Maintaining an even effort and learning to rely on perceived exertion for measuring intensity are necessary. Hal warns against trying to go hard up hills, which can lead to exhaustion. He advises making up for the slow climbs on the flats and downhills.

Besides the scrapes and cuts from falling, rolling an ankle is the trail runner's most common injury. Trail runners must strengthen their ankles. Ankle exercises are imperative. Use a wobble board, Bosu, etc., for developing balance and stability. Balancing on one leg will help with developing the stability needed for the uneven terrain and precarious footing. Additional exercises that are important for trail runners include quadriceps, core, and hip exercises (see Chapter 12).

Bicycling is great cross-training for trail running. The bike will increase your fitness, endurance, and leg strength.

How much training on trails is necessary in preparation for trail races? Hal said that when he lived in Colorado he was doing about 20 percent of his training on trails and the rest on roads. Moving to Oregon reversed that and he now does 90 percent of his training on trails. Hal says the more the better. That advice is consistent with the principle of specificity. He agreed that track repeats and long tempo runs are beneficial and can be done on the track and roads, while doing long runs on the trails. He says that's a good combination for maintaining fitness and trail endurance. This combination is especially good because many runners want to continue doing road races as well as trail runs. Hal also likes to do fartleks—fast running segments for an unspecified time or distance—on the trails.

Hal highly recommends wearing trail shoes. He points out that they provide better traction, protection with toe bumpers, and stability for lateral movements. Also the shoe uppers are built to last longer against the beating they take on the trails.

The softer impact of trails is easier on the lower body, but the likelihood of falling is much greater than with road running. The injuries are more frequently acute, rather than chronic. Trail runners must stay focused and look about 5 feet ahead at all times. If you relax or divert your attention from the trail, you fall. Falling *is* a part of trail running.

At FIRST, we are discovering that runners today are seeking varied experiences. We are not opposed to participation in a wide variety of activities, but runners must know that they may not be able to obtain their optimal performances with activities that don't necessarily complement each other.

TRIATHLON TRAINING

Scott Murr has competed in more than a hundred triathlons and has coached many triathletes, including Furman University's triathlon team. He has provided advice and recommendations for how to adapt the FIRST **3plus2** training program for triathlons. Below are Scott's recommendations in his words:

I think the FIRST training approach can be effective for triathletes. I do not know of a triathlon or cycle training program that targets the key physiological variables by workout, although it certainly makes sense that triathletes should configure their training that way.

It has been my experience that runners who are considering a triathlon want to maintain their running while simply adding swimming and cycling. These runners do not want to sacrifice their run training as they train for a triathlon. Bill and I discovered in the mid-'80s that our running performance did not decline as we shifted our training toward less running and more triathlon-specific training, eventually leading to this book.

Because there are so many variables, we have not created modified training tables for triathletes; technique and skill level are an issue with swimming, and measuring effort on the bike is problematic. Although, with the increased popularity of power meters, that could change soon.

While the swimming component of the triathlon is often the hardest, because it is the most technique-oriented activity of the three activities, it is also the shortest in both distance and time, and luckily comes first when you are freshest. Back in the '80s when I started in the sport, my swimming was weak and my strategy was "survive the swim, then race like hell."

For runners interested in completing a sprint-distance triathlon, I would suggest that they swim twice a week. Most runners who want to do a triathlon typically have a good aerobic fitness base but may not be skilled swimmers. Consequently, I think runners who are training for a triathlon need to spend a third of their time in the water performing drills to help improve their stroke technique. There are numerous resources that offer good descriptions of the basic swim drills. Runners need to practice these drills. They will help your form improve quickly if done regularly.

From my 20-year experience in the sport, I feel that the ability to run after the bike leg is as much a function of cycling training as it is of run training. Therefore, I think a runner interested in completing a sprint-distance triathlon would need to complete three bike workouts a week.

For runners interested in doing triathlons, I would suggest that they buy a road bike, rather than a triathlon bike. A road bike not only works well with the **3plus2** cross-training but can easily be configured for a tri-athlon by the simple addition of aero-bars.

I tend to think runners and triathletes should train for their event based on their current run fitness, not their triathlon run time or pace. As a runner who transitioned to the triathlon, I have found that my triathlon run times are about 10 percent slower than my open road race times.

Typically, most triathlons take place from May through October. I tend to focus on my running October through February. I start getting more focused on my cycling and swimming in March.

Here is my basic training schedule from October through February as I prepare for a spring running race.

RUN-FOCUSED TRAINING

MONDAY	30–45 minutes easy swimming or easy cycling
TUESDAY	Run (track repeats), strength training, 30 minutes easy spinning
WEDNESDAY	45–60 minutes hike (moderate-hard effort)
THURSDAY	Run (tempo effort), 30 minutes easy spinning, strength training
FRIDAY	Swim (long)
SATURDAY	Run (long)
SUNDAY	60 minutes easy spinning

This sequencing helps make the shift to a triathlon-training focus pretty manageable. I also realize that this schedule means exercising every day. While I do exercise most days, inevitably life interrupts and I miss a day. I feel that consistency in training is the key to completing a triathlon.

Yet I also think that missing a workout every now and then is not going to sabotage my training. So I don't plan a day off, but if I miss one, I'm okay with that.

Here is the basic training schedule I use as I change gears for triathlon preparation.

TRIATHLON-BASED (POSTRUN-FOCUSED) TRAINING

MONDAY	Swim (short and fast repeats)
TUESDAY	Run (track repeats), strength training, bike (easy)
WEDNESDAY	Swim (mid-distance, tempo effort) or bike (moderate-hard effort)
THURSDAY	Run (tempo effort), bike (easy-moderate effort)
FRIDAY	Swim (long) or bike (easy), strength training
SATURDAY	Bike (long)
SUNDAY	Run (long)

As FIRST suggests in the training plans for a running race, I may focus on one or two triathlons a year. So here is how I sequence my training during the 8 weeks leading up to a triathlon.

TRIATHLON PEAK (FINAL 8 WEEKS) TRAINING

MONDAY	Swim (short and fast repeats), strength training
TUESDAY	Bike (moderate-hard effort with repeats), easy transition run (~20 minutes)
WEDNESDAY	Swim (mid-distance, tempo effort), bike (easy but longer)
THURSDAY	Run (tempo effort), bike (~20 min. tempo effort)
FRIDAY	Swim (long), strength training (optional)
SATURDAY	Bike (long), easy transition run (~30 minutes)
SUNDAY	Run (long)

REAL RUNNER REPORT

I wanted to take the time to thank you for designing and publishing the most important book I've read in the past 10 years of racing. The FIRST training program changed the way I train for marathons and is now giving me a realistic opportunity to qualify for Boston.

I'm 41 years old and have been a competitive bike racer for 14 years and didn't start running marathons until 3 years ago. I followed different plans for the four marathons I've run and had limited success.

Before the ING New York City Marathon on November 7 my PR was a 3:53 at the Marine Corps Marathon in DC. But thanks to the *focus* and the *science* behind your plan I was able to PR at one of the more difficult marathons for many reasons. The long runs at given time goals was the key for me. The ease with which I ran New York and my results were astounding to me. My time in New York was a 3:35, a PR by 17 minutes!! I already have my plan laid out for my next marathon where I hope to get closer to my BQ time

Keith Slyman
System Integration Specialist
United Business Systems
Fairfield, New Jersey

Of course strength training is important. I do strength training year-round (except the 2 weeks leading up to a race). The exercises in this book are the ones that I include in my training program. I have done 12 Ironman races (6 in Kona) and the above schedules are basically the ones I have followed.

A Note on Training for an Ironman-Distance Triathlon

An Ironman-distance triathlon is a real challenge but can be managed with a smart and consistent training program. Is this something I would recommend? Only if you are genuinely motivated to do it. An alternative to the full distance of the 140.6-mile Ironman is the popular 70.3-mile half-Ironman, which can be more readily accomplished.

Just as you can approximately predict someone's marathon time from his or her 5K, 10K, or half-marathon times, you can make the same

---

REAL RUNNER REPORT

To whom it may concern,

In September 2009 I ran the Louisville City of Parks Marathon in 3:09:23, which qualified me for Boston. After qualifying I wanted to change my training approach. A friend of mine had your book sitting in the backseat of his car. While driving to our destination I skimmed through the book and was intrigued. Later that week I purchased your book and read it cover to cover.

Following your schedule for the 3:10 qualifying time, I not only felt better throughout my training but I ran a 3:03:23 in Boston!!! Your book is absolutely amazing. I have told all my friends about this training schedule and will continue to use it for all other future marathons. I was a bit of a skeptic at first because I felt I wasn't running enough throughout the week. But I stuck with the schedule. On my off-days I rode a bike for 45 to 60 minutes.

I cannot thank you enough for this amazing tool. My new goal/challenge is to break the 3-hour mark. Though the hills at Boston are no laughing matter, I believe this is very obtainable.

Eric Harshman
Assistant Groundskeeper for the Louisville Bats,
Triple A affiliate of the Cincinnati Reds
Louisville, Kentucky

---

approximation for someone's Ironman time from his or her half-Ironman times and Olympic-distance time.

To get an idea of your Ironman-distance triathlon time, take your half-Ironman time and multiply it by 2.2 to 2.4 to predict your Ironman time. Although a half-Ironman is the better predictor, you can also take your Olympic-distance time and multiply it by 4.7 to 5.0. This gives you a range where you might finish an Ironman with the appropriate training to go the distance.

CHAPTER 15

THE ROAD TO BOSTON
IS STEEPER

We receive many messages from runners asking us to help them qualify for Boston, the oldest and most prestigious American marathon. After all, running through a corridor of adoring fans for 26.2 miles is an exhilarating experience. FIRST has received hundreds of appreciative messages from Boston qualifiers.

The road to Boston has become a little steeper with the more stringent qualifying standards set for 2013. Thus we have developed new Boston training plans for each male and female age group. Each plan begins with our criteria for helping you determine if you have a realistic chance of meeting the standard, which are specific to your age and sex. You must qualify in a certified marathon.

Trying to qualify for Boston probably causes more poor marathon performances and injuries than any other goal set by runners. You might train for a too-ambitious finish time or you'll run too fast at the beginning of the race. Invariably, you'll suffer through the last half of the race, slowing considerably, and finish in a time slower than what your training predicted.

However, we believe that there is nothing more thrilling in the sport of running than the Boston Marathon. For that reason, we understand why runners are willing to risk a poor marathon experience and even injury to qualify. With that in mind, below you'll find a program that will let you know if Boston is realistic and a detailed training program that will lead to a Boston bib on Patriots' Day.

How do marathoners know if their Boston qualifying times are realistic goals? Meeting the time standard, like meeting your personal goal time in any marathon, requires being properly trained for the 26.2-mile distance and having a lot of factors—personal and external—favorable on race day. Fortunately, there are some criteria that marathoners can use to determine whether they are ready for a qualifying attempt.

Judge whether your goal is realistic by taking your finish times from 5K, 10K, or half-marathon races and see if you meet our criteria for your Boston qualifying time. **Note: The half-marathon is the best predictor.** FIRST provides another method for determining if your goal is realistic—can you run all three specified workouts for your Boston target time in the same week?

Beginning on page 210, there are 16 sets of criteria and 16 training programs, one to match each Boston qualifying time. Young and old, male and female, you'll find a program for you. Meet the criteria (metric equivalents appear in parentheses), follow the program, and look for us in Hopkinton, Massachusetts! My goal of completing Boston in each decade of my life—20s, 30s, 40s, 50s, 60s—is still on course. The once-a-decade exhilaration is sufficient to keep me motivated to continue training through the next 10 years.

THOUGHTS ON MARATHON TRAINING

Marathons provide us with an opportunity to challenge ourselves with a difficult goal that requires a dedication of time and effort spanning months. We must remember to enjoy the journey. The marathon itself lasts only a few hours, but the anticipation is spread over several months. The enjoyment that I get from having a focus for 4 months leads me to submit a marathon entry year after year. The weekend long runs give runners concrete evidence of how they are getting stronger week after week as the distance of the long runs increases. Having a goal that can be visualized during those 16 weeks provides an incentive for focused training as well as anticipation and trepidation as the race draws near.

Marathoners often share marathon training with a friend or friends. Training partners develop deep friendships, one of the benefits of running. Meeting a challenge with a friend makes it even more special. The social aspect of marathoning clearly has contributed to the tremendous growth in marathon participation.

I have run 38 marathons, 27 of them with my brother, Don. We have trained and raced together for more than 35 years. Our race times are nearly identical and we never know which of us is going to cross the finish line first. We usually run side by side until one of us pulls away near the end. We truly race with each other as much as we race against each other. We develop our racing strategy together and help pace each other in races. However, we also try to push each other. It's ideal to have a running partner who pulls you along with encouragement until the finish line is in sight when it's every man for himself.

Of course, I am doubly blessed with good training partners. Coauthor Scott Murr and I have shared more than 4,000 training runs together. In fact, Don, Scott, and I have trained together for many years. Many of the ideas for this book and its earlier edition were developed by the three of us on training runs.

Marathoners seek special destinations. Only in a marathon can you tour the monuments of Washington, DC, by running down the middle of Constitution Avenue, tour the five boroughs of New York City and experience the cheers on First Avenue, or circle the city of Chicago running up the middle of LaSalle Street. These truly are special experiences that attract thousands of runners.

Marathoners may not always appreciate what they have accomplished when they see the finish clock at the end. Unfortunately, some runners let racing become just one more source of stress in their lives. Our focus needs to be on the process and not the outcome. The vitality that training produces is what we need to appreciate and enjoy. Of course, we like to have racing goals, but we must remember that our race times do not define us. Training seriously and accepting the results without becoming despondent provide a positive, healthy experience. Sometimes everything seems perfect and a poor performance is inexplicable. It's this uncertainty that keeps many runners returning to the marathon seeking that optimal performance. Because there aren't that many opportunities to run a great marathon—ideal weather combined with excellent training—marathoners keep returning to the roads for that race where all elements come together for the performance that meets their dream expectations. And when it happens, the finish line becomes a dream come true.

Running a marathon is an immensely gratifying accomplishment. Many runners have written to us at FIRST expressing their appreciation for providing them with training programs that enabled them to realize their goals of completing a marathon or qualifying for Boston. We hope you can use this book to meet your dream challenge. Most of all, enjoy the entire marathoning process—the preparation, the runners expo, the race-day excitement, the long run itself, and the postrace euphoria. Treat it like a big recess and play hard.

BQ for Men 18 to 34: 3:05

Qualifying for Boston is realistic if you can:

Run a 5K in 19:00; a 10K in 39:45; a half-marathon in 1:28.

If you can complete one of each of the **three** key runs in the same week:

KEY RUN #1: TRACK REPEATS
(complete one of the workouts listed below)

6 × 800 @ 2:47 with 400 recovery jog between repeats

5 × 1000 @ 3:31 with 400 recovery jog between repeats

4 × 1200 @ 4:17 with 400 recovery jog between repeats

3 × 1600 @ 5:51 with 400 recovery jog between repeats

KEY RUN #2: TEMPO RUN
(complete one of the tempo runs)

After a 1-mile warmup, complete a 3-mile run in 19:15 (1.5K warmup; 5K run in 19:50)

After a 1-mile warmup, complete a 5-mile run in 33:15 (1.5K warmup; 8K run in 33:05)

After a 1-mile warmup, complete an 8-mile run in 56:12 (1.5K warmup; 13K run in 55:40)

KEY RUN #3: LONG RUN

Complete a 15- to 20-mile run @ 7:28/mile pace (24K to 32K run @ 4:38/kilometer pace)

3:05 Boston Marathon Training Plan

RI = Rest Interval; which may be a timed rest/recovery interval or a distance that you walk/jog. Key Run #1 always begins with a 10- to 20-minute warmup and ends with a 10-minute cooldown.

Metric workout equivalents appear in bold italics.

WEEK	KEY RUN #1	KEY RUN #2	KEY RUN #3
16	3 × 1600 in 5:51 (400 RI)	2 miles *(3K)* easy 2 miles at 6:24 *(3K at 3:58)* 2 miles *(3K)* easy	13 miles at 7:33 *(21K at 4:42)*
15	4 × 800 in 2:47 (2 min RI)	1 mile *(1.5K)* easy 5 miles at 7:03 *(8K at 4:23)* 1 mile *(1.5K)* easy	15 miles at 7:48 *(24K at 4:51)*
14	1200 in 4:17 (200 RI) 1000 in 3:31 (200 RI) 800 in 2:47 (200 RI) 600 in 2:05 (200 RI) 400 in 1:22 (200 RI)	1 mile *(1.5K)* easy 5 miles at 6:54 *(8K at 4:17)* 1 mile *(1.5K)* easy	17 miles at 7:48 *(27K at 4:51)*
13	5 × 1000 in 3:31 (400 RI)	1 mile *(1.5K)* easy 4 miles at 6:39 *(6.5K at 4:08)* 1 mile *(1.5K)* easy	20 miles at 8:03 *(32K at 5:00)*
12	3 × 1600 in 5:51 (400 RI)	2 miles *(3K)* easy 3 miles at 6:24 *(5K at 3:58)* 1 mile *(1.5K)* easy	18 miles at 7:48 *(29K at 4:51)*
11	2 × 1200 in 4:17 (2 min RI); 4 × 800 in 2:47 (2 min RI)	1 mile *(1.5K)* easy 5 miles at 6:39 *(8K at 4:08)* 1 mile *(1.5K)* easy	20 miles at 7:48 *(32K at 4:51)*
10	6 × 800 in 2:47 (90 sec RI)	1 mile *(1.5K)* easy 6 miles at 6:54 *(10K at 4:17)* 1 mile *(1.5K)* easy	13 miles at 7:18 *(21K at 4:32)*
9	2 × (6 × 400 in 1:22) (90 sec RI) (2 min 30 sec RI between sets)	2 miles *(3K)* easy 3 miles at 6:24 *(5K at 3:58)* 1 mile *(1.5K)* easy	18 miles at 7:33 *(29K at 4:42)*
8	2 × 1600 in 5:51 (60 sec RI) 2 × 800 in 2:47 (60 sec RI)	1 mile *(1.5K)* easy 4 miles at 6:39 *(6.5K at 4:08)* 1 mile *(1.5K)* easy	20 miles at 7:33 *(32K at 4:42)*
7	3 × (2 × 1200 in 4:17) (2 min RI) (4 min RI between sets)	10 min warmup 10 miles at 7:03 *(16K at 4:23)* 10 min cooldown	15 miles at 7:23 *(24K at 4:35)*
6	1000 in 3:31; 2000 in 7:24; 1000 in 3:31; 1000 in 3:31 (400 RI)	1 mile *(1.5K)* easy 5 miles at 7:03 *(8K at 4:23)* 1 mile *(1.5K)* easy	20 miles at 7:33 *(32K at 4:42)*

WEEK	KEY RUN #1	KEY RUN #2	KEY RUN #3
5	3 × 1600 in 5:51 (400 RI)	10 min warmup 10 miles at 7:03 *(16K at 4:23)* 10 min cooldown	15 miles at 7:18 *(24K at 4:32)*
4	10 × 400 in 1:22 (400 RI)	10 min warmup 8 miles at 7:03 *(13K at 4:23)* 10 min cooldown	20 miles at 7:18 *(32K at 4:32)*
3	8 × 800 in 2:47 (90 sec RI)	1 mile *(1.5K)* easy 5 miles at 6:39 *(8K at 4:08)* 1 mile *(1.5K)* easy	13 miles at 7:03 *(21K at 4:23)*
2	5 × 1000 in 3:31 (400 RI)	2 miles *(3K)* easy 3 miles at 6:24 *(5K at 3:58)* 1 mile *(1.5K)* easy	10 miles at 7:03 *(16K at 4:23)*
1	6 × 400 in 1:22 (400 RI)	10 min warmup 3 miles at 7:03 *(5K at 4:23)* 10-minute cooldown	MARATHON 26.2 miles at 7:03 *(42.2K at 4:23)*

BQ for Men 35 to 39: 3:10

Qualifying for Boston is realistic if you can:

Run a 5K in 19:30; a 10K in 40:50; a half-marathon in 1:30:25.

If you can complete one of each of the **three** key runs in the **same** week:

KEY RUN #1: TRACK REPEATS
(complete one of the workouts listed below)

6 × 800 @ 2:52 with 400 recovery jog between repeats

5 × 1000 @ 3:37 with 400 recovery jog between repeats

4 × 1200 @ 4:24 with 400 recovery jog between repeats

3 × 1600 @ 6:01 with 400 recovery jog between repeats

KEY RUN #2: TEMPO RUN
(complete one of the tempo runs)

After a 1-mile warmup, complete a 3-mile run in 19:45 (1.5K warmup; 5K run in 20:20)

After a 1-mile warmup, complete a 5-mile run in 34:10 (1.5K warmup; 8K run in 33:52)

After a 1-mile warmup, complete an 8-mile run in 56:30 (1.5K warmup; 13K run in 57:00)

KEY RUN #3: LONG RUN

Complete a 15- to 20-mile run @ 7:40/mile pace (24K to 32K @ 4:45/ kilometer pace)

3:10 Boston Marathon Training Plan

RI = Rest Interval; which may be a timed rest/recovery interval or a distance that you walk/jog.
Key Run #1 always begins with a 10- to 20-minute warmup and ends with a 10-minute cooldown.
Metric workout equivalents appear in bold italics.

WEEK	KEY RUN #1	KEY RUN #2	KEY RUN #3
16	3 × 1600 in 6:01 (400 RI)	2 miles *(3K)* easy 2 miles at 6:34 *(3K at 4:04)* 2 miles *(3K)* easy	13 miles at 7:44 *(21K at 4:49)*
15	4 × 800 in 2:52 (2 min RI)	1 mile *(1.5K)* easy 5 miles at 7:14 *(8K at 4:30)* 1 mile *(1.5K)* easy	15 miles at 7:59 *(24K at 4:58)*
14	1200 in 4:24 (200 RI) 1000 in 3:37 (200 RI) 800 in 2:52 (200 RI) 600 in 2:08 (200 RI) 400 in 1:24 (200 RI)	1 mile *(1.5K)* easy 5 miles at 7:04 *(8K at 4:23)* 1 mile *(1.5K)* easy	17 miles at 7:59 *(27K at 4:58)*
13	5 × 1000 in 3:37 (400 RI)	1 mile *(1.5K)* easy 4 miles at 6:49 *(6.5K at 4:14)* 1 mile *(1.5K)* easy	20 miles at 8:14 *(32K at 5:07)*
12	3 × 1600 in 6:01 (400 RI)	2 miles *(3K)* easy 3 miles at 6:34 *(5K at 4:04)* 1 mile *(1.5K)* easy	18 miles at 7:59 *(29K at 4:58)*
11	2 × 1200 in 4:24 (2 min RI) 4 × 800 in 2:52 (2 min RI)	1 mile *(1.5K)* easy 5 miles at 6:49 *(8K at 4:14)* 1 mile *(1.5K)* easy	20 miles at 7:59 *(32K at 4:58)*
10	6 × 800 in 2:52 (90 sec RI)	1 mile *(1.5K)* easy 6 miles at 7:04 *(10K at 4:23)* 1 mile *(1.5K)* easy	13 miles at 7:29 *(21K at 4:39)*
9	2 × (6 × 400 in 1:24) (90 sec RI) (2 min 30 sec RI between sets)	2 miles *(3K)* easy 3 miles at 6:34 *(5K at 4:04)* 1 mile *(1.5K)* easy	18 miles at 7:44 *(29K at 4:49)*
8	2 × 1600 in 6:01 (60 sec RI) 2 × 800 in 2:52 (60 sec RI)	1 mile *(1.5K)* easy 4 miles at 6:49 *(6.5K at 4:14)* 1 mile *(1.5K)* easy	20 miles at 7:44 *(32K at 4:49)*
7	3 × (2 × 1200 in 4:24) (2 min RI) (4 min RI between sets)	10 min warmup 10 miles at 7:14 *(16K at 4:30)* 10 min cooldown	15 miles at 7:34 *(24K at 4:42)*
6	1000 in 3:37; 2000 in 7:36; 1000 in 3:37; 1000 in 3:37 (400 RI)	1 mile *(1.5K)* easy 5 miles at 7:14 *(8K at 4:30)* 1 mile *(1.5K)* easy	20 miles at 7:44 *(32K at 4:49)*

WEEK	KEY RUN #1	KEY RUN #2	KEY RUN #3
5	3 x 1600 in 6:01 (400 RI)	10 min warmup 10 miles at 7:14 *(16K at 4:30)* 10 min cooldown	15 miles at 7:29 *(24K at 4:39)*
4	10 x 400 in 1:24 (400 RI)	10 min warmup 8 miles at 7:14 *(13K at 4:30)* 10 min cooldown	20 miles at 7:29 *(32K at 4:39)*
3	8 x 800 in 2:52 (90 sec RI)	1 mile *(1.5K)* easy 5 miles at 6:49 *(8K at 4:14)* 1 mile *(1.5K)* easy	13 miles at 7:14 *(21K at 4:30)*
2	5 x 1000 in 3:37 (400 RI)	2 miles *(3K)* easy 3 miles at 6:34 *(5K at 4:04)* 1 mile *(1.5K)* easy	10 miles at 7:14 *(16K at 4:30)*
1	6 x 400 in 1:24 (400 RI)	10 min warmup 3 miles at 7:14 *(5K at 4:30)* 10 min cooldown	MARATHON 26.2 miles at 7:14 *(42.2K at 4:30)*

BQ for Men 40 to 44: 3:15

Qualifying for Boston is realistic if you can:

Run a 5K in 20:05; a 10K in 42:00; a half-marathon in 1:33:30.

If you can complete one of each of the **three** key runs in the same week.

KEY RUN #1: TRACK REPEATS
(complete one of the workouts listed below)

6 × 800 @ 2:58 with 400 recovery jog between repeats

5 × 1000 @ 3:44 with 400 recovery jog between repeats

4 × 1200 @ 4:33 with 400 recovery jog between repeats

3 × 1600 @ 6:12 with 400 recovery jog between repeats

KEY RUN #2: TEMPO RUN
(complete one of the tempo runs)

After a 1-mile warmup, complete a 3-mile run in 20:15 (1.5K warmup; 5K run in 20:55)

After a 1-mile warmup, complete a 5-mile run in 35:00 (1.5K warmup; 8K run in 34:50)

After a 1-mile warmup, complete an 8-mile run in 58:00 (1.5K warmup; 13K run in 56:30)

KEY RUN #3: LONG RUN

Complete a 15- to 20-mile run @ 7:50/mile pace (24K to 32K run @ 4:53/kilometer pace)

3:15 Boston Marathon Training Plan

RI = Rest Interval; which may be a timed rest/recovery interval or a distance that you walk/jog. Key Run #1 always begins with a 10- to 20-minute warmup and ends with a 10-minute cooldown.

Metric workout equivalents appear in bold italics.

WEEK	KEY RUN #1	KEY RUN #2	KEY RUN #3
16	3 × 1600 in 6:12 (400 RI)	2 miles *(3K)* easy 2 miles at 6:45 *(3K at 4:11)* 2 miles *(3K)* easy	13 miles at 7:56 *(21K at 4:57)*
15	4 × 800 in 2:58 (2 min RI)	1 mile *(1.5K)* easy 5 miles at 7:26 *(8K at 4:37)* 1 mile *(1.5K)* easy	15 miles at 8:11 *(24K at 5:06)*
14	1200 in 4:33 (200 RI) 1000 in 3:44 (200 RI) 800 in 2:58 (200 RI) 600 in 2:13 (200 RI) 400 in 1:27 (200 RI)	1 mile *(1.5K)* easy 5 miles at 7:15 *(8K at 4:30)* 1 mile *(1.5K)* easy	17 miles at 8:11 *(27K at 5:06)*
13	5 × 1000 in 3:44 (400 RI)	1 mile *(1.5K)* easy 4 miles at 7:00 *(6.5K at 4:21)* 1 mile *(1.5K)* easy	20 miles at 8:26 *(32K at 5:15)*
12	3 × 1600 in 6:12 (400 RI)	2 miles *(3K)* easy 3 miles at 6:45 *(5K at 4:11)* 1 mile *(1.5K)* easy	18 miles at 8:11 *(29K at 5:06)*
11	2 × 1200 in 4:33 (2 min RI) 4 × 800 in 2:58 (2 min RI)	1 mile *(1.5K)* easy 5 miles at 7:00 *(8K at 4:21)* 1 mile *(1.5K)* easy	20 miles at 8:11 *(32K at 5:06)*
10	6 × 800 in 2:58 (90 sec RI)	1 mile *(1.5K)* easy 6 miles at 7:15 *(10K at 4:30)* 1 mile *(1.5K)* easy	13 miles at 7:41 *(21K at 4:47)*
9	2 × (6 × 400 in 1:27) (90 sec RI) (2 min 30 sec RI between sets)	2 miles *(3K)* easy 3 miles at 6:45 *(5K at 4:11)* 1 mile *(1.5K)* easy	18 miles at 7:56 *(29K at 4:57)*
8	2 × 1600 in 6:12 (60 sec RI) 2 × 800 in 2:58 (60 sec RI)	1 mile *(1.5K)* easy 4 miles at 7:00 *(6.5K at 4:21)* 1 mile *(1.5K)* easy	20 miles at 7:56 *(32K at 4:57)*
7	3 × (2 × 1200 in 4:33) (2 min RI) (4 min RI between sets)	10 min warmup 10 miles at 7:26 *(16K at 4:37)* 10 min cooldown	15 miles at 7:46 *(24K at 4:50)*
6	1000 in 3:44; 2000 in 7:50; 1000 in 3:44; 1000 in 3:44 (400 RI)	1 mile *(1.5K)* easy 5 miles at 7:26 *(8K at 4:37)* 1 mile *(1.5K)* easy	20 miles at 7:56 *(32K at 4:57)*

WEEK	KEY RUN #1	KEY RUN #2	KEY RUN #3
5	3 × 1600 in 6:12 (400 RI)	10 min warmup 10 miles at 7:26 *(16K at 4:37)* 10 min cooldown	15 miles at 7:41 *(24K at 4:47)*
4	10 × 400 in 1:27 (400 RI)	10 min warmup 8 miles at 7:26 *(13K at 4:37)* 10 min cooldown	20 miles at 7:41 *(32K at 4:47)*
3	8 × 800 in 2:58 (90 sec RI)	1 mile *(1.5K)* easy 5 miles at 7:00 *(8K at 4:21)* 1 mile *(1.5K)* easy	13 miles at 7:26 *(21K at 4:37)*
2	5 × 1000 in 3:44 (400 RI)	2 miles *(3K)* easy 3 miles at 6:45 *(5K at 4:11)* 1 mile *(1.5K)* easy	10 miles at 7:26 *(16K at 4:37)*
1	6 × 400 in 1:27 (400 RI)	10 min warmup 3 miles at 7:26 *(5K at 4:37)* 10 min cooldown	MARATHON 26.2 miles at 7:26 *(42.2K at 4:37)*

BQ for Men 45 to 49: 3:25

Qualifying for Boston is realistic if you can:

> Run a 5K in 21:05; a 10K in 44:06; a half-marathon in 1:38:00.
>
> If you can complete one of each of the **three** key runs in the **same** week:

KEY RUN #1: TRACK REPEATS
(complete one of the workouts listed below)

> 6 × 800 @ 3:08 with 400 recovery jog between repeats
>
> 5 × 1000 @ 3:56 with 400 recovery jog between repeats
>
> 4 × 1200 @ 4:47 with 400 recovery jog between repeats
>
> 3 × 1600 @ 6:31 with 400 recovery jog between repeats

KEY WORKOUT #2: TEMPO RUN
(complete one of the tempo runs)

> After a 1-mile warmup, complete a 3-mile run in 21:15 (1.5K warmup: 5K run in 21:55)
>
> After a 1-mile warmup, complete a 5-mile run in 36:30 (1.5K warmup; 8K run in 36:24)
>
> After a 1-mile warmup, complete an 8-mile run in 60:24 (1.5K warmup; 13K run in 61:06)

KEY WORKOUT #3: LONG RUN

> Complete a 15- to 20-mile run @ 8:15/mile pace (24K to 32K run @ 5:07/kilometer pace)

3:25 Boston Marathon Training Plan

RI = Rest Interval; which may be a timed rest/recovery interval or a distance that you walk/jog
Key Run #1 always begins with a 10- to 20-minute warmup and ends with a 10-minute cooldown
Metric workout equivalents appear in bold italics.

WEEK	KEY RUN #1	KEY RUN #2	KEY RUN #3
16	3 × 1600 in 6:31 (400 RI)	2 miles *(3K)* easy 2 miles at 7:04 *(3K at 4:23)* 2 miles *(3K)* easy	13 miles at 8:19 *(21K at 5:10)*
15	4 × 800 in 3:08 (2 min RI)	1 mile *(1.5K)* easy 5 miles at 7:49 *(8K at 4:51)* 1 mile *(1.5K)* easy	15 miles at 8:34 *(24K at 5:19)*
14	1200 in 4:47 (200 RI) 1000 in 3:56 (200 RI) 800 in 3:08 (200 RI) 600 in 2:20 (200 RI) 400 in 1:32 (200 RI)	1 mile *(1.5K)* easy 5 miles at 7:34 *(8K at 4:42)* 1 mile *(1.5K)* easy	17 miles at 8:34 *(27K at 5:19)*
13	5 × 1000 in 3:56 (400 RI)	1 mile *(1.5K)* easy 4 miles at 7:19 *(6.5K at 4:33)* 1 mile *(1.5K)* easy	20 miles at 8:49 *(32K at 5:28)*
12	3 × 1600 in 6:31 (400 RI)	2 miles *(3K)* easy 3 miles at 7:04 *(5K at 4:23)* 1 mile *(1.5K)* easy	18 miles at 8:34 *(29K at 5:19)*
11	2 × 1200 in 4:47 (2 min RI) 4 × 800 in 3:08 (2 min RI)	1 mile *(1.5K)* easy 5 miles at 7:19 *(8K at 4:33)* 1 mile *(1.5K)* easy	20 miles at 8:34 *(32K at 5:19)*
10	6 × 800 in 3:08 (90 sec RI)	1 mile *(1.5K)* easy 6 miles at 7:34 *(10K at 4:42)* 1 mile *(1.5K)* easy	13 miles at 8:04 *(21K at 5:00)*
9	2 × (6 × 400 in 1:32) (90 sec RI) (2 min 30 sec RI between sets)	2 miles *(3K)* easy 3 miles at 7:04 *(5K at 4:23)* 1 mile *(1.5K)* easy	18 miles at 8:19 *(29K at 5:10)*
8	2 × 1600 in 6:31 (60 sec RI) 2 × 800 in 3:08 (60 sec RI)	1 mile *(1.5K)* easy 4 miles at 7:19 *(6.5K at 4:33)* 1 mile *(1.5K)* easy	20 miles at 8:19 *(32K at 5:10)*
7	3 × (2 × 1200 in 4:47) (2 min RI) (4 min RI between sets)	10 min warmup 10 miles at 7:49 *(16K at 4:51)* 10 min cooldown	15 miles at 8:09 *(24K at 5:03)*
6	1000 in 3:56; 2000 in 8:14; 1000 in 3:56; 1000 in 3:56 (400 RI)	1 mile *(1.5K)* easy 5 miles at 7:49 *(8K at 4:51)* 1 mile *(1.5K)* easy	20 miles at 8:19 *(32K at 5:10)*

WEEK	KEY RUN #1	KEY RUN #2	KEY RUN #3
5	3 × 1600 in 6:31 (400 RI)	10 min warmup 10 miles at 7:49 *(16K at 4:51)* 10 min cooldown	15 miles at 8:04 *(24K at 5:00)*
4	10 × 400 in 1:32 (400 RI)	10 min warmup 8 miles at 7:49 *(13K at 4:51)* 10 min cooldown	20 miles at 8:04 *(32K at 5:00)*
3	8 × 800 in 3:08 (90 sec RI)	1 mile *(1.5K)* easy 5 miles at 7:19 *(8K at 4:33)* 1 mile *(1.5K)* easy	13 miles at 7:49 *(21K at 4:51)*
2	5 × 1000 in 3:56 (400 RI)	2 miles *(3K)* easy 3 miles at 7:04 *(5K at 4:23)* 1 mile *(1.5K)* easy	10 miles at 7:49 *(16K at 4:51)*
1	6 × 400 in 1:32 (400 RI)	10 min warmup 3 miles at 7:49 *(5K at 4:51)* 10 min cooldown	MARATHON 26.2 miles at 7:49 *(42.2K at 4:51)*

BQ for Men 50 to 54: 3:30

Qualifying for Boston is realistic if you can:

Run a 5K in 21:35; a 10K in 45:10; a half-marathon in 1:40:00.

If you can complete one of each of the **three** key runs in the **same week**:

KEY RUN #1: TRACK REPEATS
(complete one of the workouts listed below)

6 × 800 @ 3:13 with 400 recovery jog between repeats

5 × 1000 @ 4:02 with 400 recovery jog between repeats

4 × 1200 @ 4:54 with 400 recovery jog between repeats

3 × 1600 @ 6:41 with 400 recovery jog between repeats

KEY RUN #2: TEMPO RUN
(complete one of the tempo runs)

After a 1-mile warmup, complete a 3-mile run in 21:42 (1.5K warmup; 5K run in 22:25)

After a 1-mile warmup, complete a 5-mile run in 37:30 (1.5K warmup; 8K run in 37:15)

After a 1-mile warmup, complete an 8-mile run in 62:00 (1.5K warmup; 13K run in 62:24)

KEY RUN #3: LONG RUN

Complete a 15- to 20-mile run @ 8:25/mile pace (24K to 32K @ 5:15/ kilometer pace)

3:30 Boston Marathon Training Plan

RI = Rest Interval; which may be a timed rest/recovery interval or a distance that you walk/jog. Key Run #1 always begins with a 10- to 20-minute warmup and ends with a 10-minute cooldown.

Metric workout equivalents appear in bold italics.

WEEK	KEY RUN #1	KEY RUN #2	KEY RUN #3
16	3 × 1600 in 6:41 (400 RI)	2 miles *(3K)* easy 2 miles at 7:14 *(3K at 4:29)* 2 miles *(3K)* easy	13 miles at 8:30 *(21K at 5:18)*
15	4 × 800 in 3:13 (2 min RI)	1 mile *(1.5K)* easy 5 miles at 8:00 *(8K at 4:59)* 1 mile *(1.5K)* easy	15 miles at 8:45 *(24K at 5:27)*
14	1200 in 4:54 (200 RI); 1000 in 4:02 (200 RI); 800 in 3:13 (200 RI); 600 in 2:24 (200 RI); 400 in 1:34 (200 RI)	1 mile *(1.5K)* easy 5 miles at 7:44 *(8K at 4:48)* 1 mile *(1.5K)* easy	17 miles at 8:45 *(27K at 5:27)*
13	5 × 1000 in 4:02 (400 RI)	1 mile *(1.5K)* easy 4 miles at 7:29 *(6.5K at 4:39)* 1 mile *(1.5K)* easy	20 miles at 9:00 *(32K at 5:36)*
12	3 × 1600 in 6:41 (400 RI)	2 miles *(3K)* easy 3 miles at 7:14 *(5K at 4:29)* 1 mile *(1.5K)* easy	18 miles at 8:45 *(29K at 5:27)*
11	2 × 1200 in 4:54 (2 min RI);, 4 × 800 in 3:13 (2 min RI)	1 mile *(1.5K)* easy 5 miles at 7:29 *(8K at 4:39)* 1 mile *(1.5K)* easy	20 miles at 8:45 *(32K at 5:27)*
10	6 × 800 in 3:13 (90 sec RI)	1 mile *(1.5K)* easy 6 miles at 7:44 *(10K at 4:48)* 1 mile *(1.5K)* easy	13 miles at 8:15 *(21K at 5:08)*
9	2 × (6 × 400 in 1:34) (90 sec RI) (2 min 30 sec RI between sets)	2 miles *(3K)* easy 3 miles at 7:14 *(5K at 4:29)* 1 mile *(1.5K)* easy	18 miles at 8:30 *(29K at 5:18)*
8	2 × 1600 in 6:41 (60 sec RI); 2 × 800 in 3:13 (60 sec RI)	1 mile *(1.5K)* easy 4 miles at 7:29 *(6.5K at 4:39)* 1 mile *(1.5K)* easy	20 miles at 8:30 *(32K at 5:18)*
7	3 × (2 × 1200 in 4:54) (2 min RI) (4 min RI between sets)	10 min warmup 10 miles at 8:00 *(16K at 4:49)* 10 min cooldown	15 miles at 8:20 *(24K at 5:11)*
6	1000 in 4:02; 2000 in 8:26; 1000 in 4:02; 1000 in 4:02 (400 RI)	1 mile *(1.5K)* easy 5 miles at 8:00 *(8K at 4:49)* 1 mile *(1.5K)* easy	20 miles at 8:30 *(32K at 5:18)*

WEEK	KEY RUN #1	KEY RUN #2	KEY RUN #3
5	3 × 1600 in 6:41 (400 RI)	10 min warmup 10 miles at 8:00 *(16K at 4:49)* 10 min cooldown	15 miles at 8:15 *(24K at 5:08)*
4	10 × 400 in 1:34 (400 RI)	10 min warmup 8 miles at 8:00 *(13K at 4:49)* 10 min cooldown	20 miles at 8:15 *(18K at 5:08)*
3	8 × 800 in 3:13 (90 sec RI)	1 mile *(1.5K)* easy 5 miles at 7:29 *(8K at 4:39)* 1 mile *(1.5K)* easy	13 miles at 8:00 *(21K at 4:59)*
2	5 × 1000 in 4:02 (400 RI)	2 miles *(3K)* easy 3 miles at 7:14 *(5K at 4:29)* 1 mile *(1.5K)* easy	10 miles at 8:00 *(16K at 4:59)*
1	6 × 400 in 1:34 (400 RI)	10 min warmup 3 miles at 8:00 *(5K at 4:49)* 10 min cooldown	MARATHON 26.2 miles at 8:00 *(42.2K at 4:59)*

BQ for Women 18 to 34: 3:35

Qualifying for Boston is realistic if you can:

Run a 5K in 22:05; a 10K in 46:10; a half-marathon in 1:42:20.

If you can complete one of each of the **three** key runs in the **same** week:

KEY RUN #1: TRACK REPEATS
(complete one of the workouts listed below)

6 × 800 @ 3:17 with 400 recovery jog between repeats

5 × 1000 @ 4:09 with 400 recovery jog between repeats

4 × 1200 @ 5:02 with 400 recovery jog between repeats

3 × 1600 @ 6:51 with 400 recovery jog between repeats

KEY RUN #2: TEMPO RUN
(complete one of the tempo runs)

After a 1-mile warmup, complete a 3-mile run in 22:09 (1.5K warmup; 5K run in 22:55)

After a 1-mile warmup, complete a 5-mile run in 38:10 (1.5K warmup; 8K run in 38:00)

After a 1-mile warmup, complete an 8-mile run in 63:04 (1.5K warmup; 13K run in 63:42)

KEY RUN #3: LONG RUN

Complete a 15- to 20-mile run @ 8:37/mile pace (24K to 32K @ 5:20/kilometer pace)

3:35 Boston Marathon Training Plan

RI = Rest Interval; which may be a timed rest/recovery interval or a distance that you walk/jog.
Key Run #1 always begins with a 10- to 20-min warmup and ends with a 10-minute cooldown.
Metric workout equivalents appear in bold italics.

WEEK	KEY RUN #1	KEY RUN #2	KEY RUN #3
16	3 × 1600 in 6:51 (400 RI)	2 miles *(3K)* easy 2 miles at 7:23 *(3K at 4:35)* 2 miles *(3K)* easy	13 miles at 8:40 *(21K at 5:24)*
15	4 × 800 in 3:17 (2 min RI)	1 mile *(1.5K)* easy 5 miles at 8:12 *(8K at 5:05)* 1 mile *(1.5K)* easy	15 miles at 8:57 *(24K at 5:33)*
14	1200 in 5:02 (200 RI); 1000 in 4:09 (200 RI); 800 in 3:17 (200 RI); 600 in 2:27 (200 RI); 400 in 1:36 (200 RI)	1 mile *(1.5K)* easy 5 miles at 7:53 *(8K at 4:54)* 1 mile *(1.5K)* easy	17 miles at 8:57 *(27K at 5:33)*
13	5 × 1000 in 4:09 (400 RI)	1 mile *(1.5K)* easy 4 miles at 7:38 *(6.5K at 4:45)* 1 mile *(1.5K)* easy	20 miles at 9:12 *(32K at 5:42)*
12	3 × 1600 in 6:51 (400 RI)	2 miles *(3K)* easy 3 miles at 7:23 *(5K at 4:35)* 1 mile *(1.5K)* easy	18 miles at 8:57 *(29K at 5:33)*
11	2 × 1200 in 5:02 (2 min RI); 4 × 800 in 3:17 (2 min RI)	1 mile *(1.5K)* easy 5 miles at 7:38 *(8K at 4:45)* 1 mile *(1.5K)* easy	20 miles at 8:57 *(32K at 5:33)*
10	6 × 800 in 3:17 (90 sec RI)	1 mile *(1.5K)* easy 6 miles at 7:53 *(10K at 4:54)* 1 mile *(1.5K)* easy	13 miles at 8:27 *(21K at 5:14)*
9	2 × (6x 400 in 1:36) (90 sec RI) (2 min 30 sec RI between sets)	2 miles *(3K)* easy 3 miles at 7:23 *(5K at 4:35)* 1 mile *(1.5K)* easy	18 miles at 8:40 *(29K at 5:24)*
8	2 × 1600 in 6:51 (60 sec RI) 2 × 800 in 3:17 (60 sec RI)	1 mile *(1.5K)* easy 4 miles at 7:38 *(6.5K at 4:45)* 1 mile *(1.5K)* easy	20 miles at 8:40 *(32K at 5:24)*
7	3 × (2 × 1200 in 5:02) (2 min RI) (4 min RI between sets)	10 min warmup 10 miles at 8:12 *(16K at 5:05)* 10 min cooldown	15 miles at 8:32 *(24K at 5:17)*
6	1000 in 4:09; 2000 in 8:37; 1000 in 4:09; 1000 in 4:09 (400 RI)	1 mile *(1.5K)* easy 5 miles at 8:12 *(8K at 5:05)* 1 mile *(1.5K)* easy	20 miles at 8:40 *(32K at 5:24)*

WEEK	KEY RUN #1	KEY RUN #2	KEY RUN #3
5	3 x 1600 in 6:51 (400 RI)	10 min warmup 10 miles at 8:12 *(16K at 5:05)* 10 min cooldown	15 miles at 8:27 *(24K at 5:14)*
4	10 x 400 in 1:36 (400 RI)	10 min warmup 8 miles at 8:12 *(13K at 5:05)* 10 min cooldown	20 miles at 8:27 *(32K at 5:14)*
3	8 x 800 in 3:17 (90 sec RI)	1 mile *(1.5K)* easy 5 miles at 7:38 *(8K at 4:45)* 1 mile *(1.5K)* easy	13 miles at 8:12 *(21K at 5:05)*
2	5 x 1000 in 4:09 (400 RI)	2 miles *(3K)* easy 3 miles at 7:23 *(5K at 4:35)* 1 mile *(1.5K)* easy	10 miles at 8:12 *(16K at 5:05)*
1	6 x 400 in 1:36 (400 RI)	10 min warmup 3 miles at 8:12 *(5K at 5:05)* 10 min cooldown	MARATHON 26.2 miles at 8:12 *(42.2K at 5:05)*

BQ for Men 55 to 59 and Women 35 to 39: 3:40

Qualifying for Boston is realistic if you can:

Run a 5K in 22:40; a 10K in 47:25; a half-marathon in 1:45:00.

If you can complete one of each of the **three** key runs in the **same** week:

KEY RUN #1: TRACK REPEATS
(complete one of the workouts listed below)

6 × 800 @ 3:23 with 400 recovery jog between repeats

5 × 1000 @ 4:16 with 400 recovery jog between repeats

4 × 1200 @ 5:10 with 400 recovery jog between repeats

3 × 1600 @ 7:02 with 400 recovery jog between repeats

KEY RUN #2: TEMPO RUN
(complete one of the tempo runs)

After a 1-mile warmup, complete a 3-mile run in 22:45 (1.5K warmup; 5K run in 23:30)

After a 1-mile warmup, complete a 5-mile run in 39:10 (1.5K warmup; 8K run in 38:56)

After a 1-mile warmup, complete an 8-mile run in 64:40 (1.5K warmup; 13K run in 65:13)

KEY RUN #3: LONG RUN

Complete a 15- to 20-mile run @ 8:48/mile pace (24K to 32K @ 5:29/ kilometer pace)

3:40 Boston Marathon Training Plan

RI = Rest Interval; which may be a timed rest/recovery interval or a distance that you walk/jog. Key Run #1 always begins with a 10- to 20-minute warmup and ends with a 10-minute cooldown.

Metric workout equivalents appear in bold italics.

WEEK	KEY RUN #1	KEY RUN #2	KEY RUN #3
16	3 × 1600 in 7:02 (400 RI)	2 miles *(3K)* easy 2 miles at 7:35 *(3K at 4:42)* 2 miles *(3K)* easy	13 miles at 8:53 *(21K at 5:31)*
15	4 × 800 in 3:23 (2 min RI)	1 mile *(1.5K)* easy 5 miles at 8:23 *(8K at 5:14)* 1 mile *(1.5K)* easy	15 miles at 9:08 *(24K at 5:41)*
14	1200 in 5:10 (200 RI); 1000 in 4:16 (200 RI); 800 in 3:23 (200 RI); 600 in 2:31 (200 RI); 400 in 1:39 (200 RI)	1 mile *(1.5K)* easy 5 miles at 8:05 *(8K at 5:01)* 1 mile *(1.5K)* easy	17 miles at 9:08 *(27K at 5:41)*
13	5 × 1000 in 4:16 (400 RI)	1 mile *(1.5K)* easy 4 miles at 7:50 *(6.5K at 4:52)* 1 mile *(1.5K)* easy	20 miles at 9:23 *(32K at 5:50)*
12	3 × 1600 in 7:02 (400 RI)	2 miles *(3K)* easy 3 miles at 7:35 *(5K at 4:42)* 1 mile *(1.5K)* easy	18 miles at 9:08 *(29K at 5:41)*
11	2 × 1200 in 5:10 (2 min RI); 4 × 800 in 3:23 (2 min RI)	1 mile *(1.5K)* easy 5 miles at 7:50 *(8K at 4:52)* 1 mile *(1.5K)* easy	20 miles at 9:08 *(32K at 5:41)*
10	6 × 800 in 3:23 (90 sec RI)	1 mile *(1.5K)* easy 6 miles at 8:05 *(10K at 5:01)* 1 mile *(1.5K)* easy	13 miles at 8:38 *(21K at 5:22)*
9	2 × (6 × 400 in 1:39) (90 sec RI) (2 min 30 sec RI between sets)	2 miles *(3K)* easy 3 miles at 7:35 *(5K at 4:42)* 1 mile *(1.5K)* easy	18 miles at 8:53 *(29K at 5:31)*
8	2 × 1600 in 7:02 (60 sec RI) 2 × 800 in 3:23 (60 sec RI)	1 mile *(1.5K)* easy 4 miles at 7:50 *(6.5K at 4:52)* 1 mile *(1.5K)* easy	20 miles at 8:53 *(32K at 5:31)*
7	3 × (2 × 1200 in 5:10) (2 min RI) (4 min RI between sets)	10 min warmup 10 miles at 8:23 *(16K at 5:14)* 10 min cooldown	15 miles at 8:43 *(24K at 5:25)*
6	1000 in 4:16; 2000 in 8:52; 1000 in 4:16; 1000 in 4:16 (400 RI)	1 mile *(1.5K)* easy 5 miles at 8:23 *(8K at 5:14)* 1 mile *(1.5K)* easy	20 miles at 8:53 *(32K at 5:31)*

WEEK	KEY RUN #1	KEY RUN #2	KEY RUN #3
5	3 × 1600 in 7:02 (400 RI)	10 min warmup 10 miles at 8:23 *(16K at 5:14)* 10 min cooldown	15 miles at 8:38 *(24K at 5:22)*
4	10 × 400 in 1:39 (400 RI)	10 min warmup 8 miles at 8:23 *(13K at 5:14)* 10 min cooldown	20 miles at 8:38 *(32K at 5:22)*
3	8 × 800 in 3:23 (90 sec RI)	1 mile *(1.5K)* easy 5 miles at 7:50 *(8K at 4:52)* 1 mile *(1.5K)* easy	13 miles at 8:23 *(21K at 5:13)*
2	5 × 1000 in 4:16 (400 RI)	2 miles *(3K)* easy 3 miles at 7:35 *(5K at 4:42)* 1 mile *(1.5K)* easy	10 miles at 8:23 *(16K at 5:13)*
1	6 × 400 in 1:39 (400 RI)	10 min warmup 3 miles at 8:23 *(5K at 5:14)* 10 min cooldown	MARATHON 26.2 miles at 8:23 *(42.2K at 5:13)*

BQ Women 40 to 44: 3:45

Qualifying for Boston is realistic if you can:

Run a 5K in 23:10; a 10K in 48:30; a half-marathon in 1:47:25.

If you can complete one of each of the **three** key runs in the **same** week:

KEY RUN #1: TRACK REPEATS
(complete one of the workouts listed below)

6 × 800 @ 3:27 with 400 recovery jog between repeats

5 × 1000 @ 4:22 with 400 recovery jog between repeats

4 × 1200 @ 5:18 with 400 recovery jog between repeats

3 × 1600 @ 7:11 with 400 recovery jog between repeats

KEY RUN #2: TEMPO RUN
(complete one of the tempo runs)

After a 1-mile warmup, complete a 3-mile run in 23:15 (1.5K warmup; 5K run in 24:00)

After a 1-mile warmup, complete a 5-mile run in 40:00 (1.5K warmup; 8K run in 39:44)

After a 1-mile warmup, complete an 8-mile run in 66:00 (1.5K warmup; 13K run in 66:31)

KEY #3: LONG RUN

Complete a 15- to 20-mile run @ 9:00/mile pace (24K to 32K at 5:36/kilometer pace)

3:45 Boston Marathon Training Plan

RI = Rest Interval; which may be a timed rest/recovery interval or a distance that you walk/jog. Key Run #1 always begins with a 10- to 20-minute warmup and ends with a 10-minute cooldown.

Metric workout equivalents appear in bold italics.

WEEK	KEY RUN #1	KEY RUN #2	KEY RUN #3
16	3 × 1600 in 7:11 (400 RI)	2 miles *(3K)* easy 2 miles at 7:44 *(3K at 4:48)* 2 miles *(3K)* easy	13 miles at 9:05 *(21K at 5:39)*
15	4 × 800 in 3:27 (2 min RI)	1 mile *(1.5K)* easy 5 miles at 8:35 *(8K at 5:20)* 1 mile *(1.5K)* easy	15 miles at 9:20 *(24K at 5:48)*
14	1200 in 5:18 (200 RI); 1000 in 4:22 (200 RI); 800 in 3:27 (200 RI); 600 in 2:35 (200 RI); 400 in 1:42 (200 RI)	1 mile *(1.5K)* easy 5 miles at 8:14 *(8K at 5:07)* 1 mile *(1.5K)* easy	17 miles at 9:20 *(27K at 5:48)*
13	5 × 1000 in 4:22 (400 RI)	1 mile *(1.5K)* easy 4 miles at 7:59 *(6.5K at 4:58)* 1 mile *(1.5K)* easy	20 miles at 9:35 *(32K at 5:57)*
12	3 × 1600 in 7:11 (400 RI)	2 miles *(3K)* easy 3 miles at 7:44 *(5K at 4:48)* 1 mile *(1.5K)* easy	18 miles at 9:20 *(29K at 5:48)*
11	2 × 1200 in 5:18 (2 min RI); 4 × 800 in 3:27 (2 min RI)	1 mile *(1.5K)* easy 5 miles at 7:59 *(8K at 4:58)* 1 mile *(1.5K)* easy	20 miles at 9:20 *(32K at 5:48)*
10	6 × 800 in 3:27 (90 sec RI)	1 mile *(1.5K)* easy 6 miles at 8:14 *(10K at 5:07)* 1 mile *(1.5K)* easy	13 miles at 8:50 *(21K at 5:39)*
9	2 × (6 × 400 in 1:42) (90 sec RI) (2 min 30 sec RI between sets)	2 miles *(3K)* easy 3 miles at 7:44 *(5K at 4:48)* 1 mile *(1.5K)* easy	18 miles at 9:05 *(29K at 5:39)*
8	2 × 1600 in 7:11 (60 sec RI) 2 × 800 in 3:27 (60 sec RI)	1 mile *(1.5K)* easy 4 miles at 7:59 *(6.5K at 4:58)* 1 mile *(1.5K)* easy	20 miles at 9:05 *(32K at 5:39)*
7	3 × (2 × 1200 in 5:18) (2 min RI) (4 min RI between sets)	10 min warmup 10 miles at 8:35 *(16K at 5:20)* 10 min cooldown	15 miles at 8:55 *(24K at 5:32)*
6	1000 in 4:22; 2000 in 9:04; 1000 in 4:22; 1000 in 4:22 (400 RI)	1 mile *(1.5K)* easy 5 miles at 8:35 *(8K at 5:20)* 1 mile *(1.5K)* easy	20 miles at 9:05 *(32K at 5:39)*

WEEK	KEY RUN #1	KEY RUN #2	KEY RUN #3
5	3 × 1600 in 7:11 (400 RI)	10 min warmup 10 miles at 8:35 *(16K at 5:20)* 10 min cooldown	15 miles at 8:50 *(24K at 5:29)*
4	10 × 400 in 1:42 (400 RI)	10 min warmup 8 miles at 8:35 *(13K at 5:20)* 10 min cooldown	20 miles at 8:50 *(32K at 5:29)*
3	8 × 800 in 3:27 (90 sec RI)	1 mile *(1.5K)* easy 5 miles at 7:59 *(8K at 4:58)* 1 mile *(1.5K)* easy	13 miles at 8:35 *(21K at 5:20)*
2	5 × 1000 in 4:22 (400 RI)	2 miles *(3K)* easy 3 miles at 7:44 *(5K at 4:48)* 1 mile *(1.5K)* easy	10 miles at 8:35 *(16K at 5:20)*
1	6 × 400 in 1:42 (400 RI)	10 min warmup 3 miles at 8:35 *(5K at 5:20)* 10 min cooldown	MARATHON 26.2 miles at 8:35 *(42.2K at 5:20)*

BQ for Men 60 to 64 and Women 45 to 49: 3:55

Qualifying for Boston is realistic if you can:

Run a 5K in 24:10; a 10K in 50:34; a half-marathon in 1:52:00.

If you can complete one of each of the **three key runs** in the same week:

KEY RUN #1: TRACK REPEATS
(complete one of the workouts listed below)

6 × 800 @ 3:37 with 400 recovery jog between repeats

5 × 1000 @ 4:34 with 400 recovery jog between repeats

4 × 1200 @ 5:32 with 400 recovery jog between repeats

3 × 1600 @ 7:30 with 400 recovery jog between repeats

KEY RUN #2: TEMPO RUN
(complete one of the tempo runs)

After a 1-mile warmup, complete a 3-mile run in 24:12 (1.5K warmup; 5K run in 25:00)

After a 1-mile warmup, complete a 5-mile run in 41:35 (1.5K warmup; 8K run in 41:20)

After a 1-mile warmup, complete an 8-mile run in 68:32 (1.5K warmup; 13K run in 69:07)

KEY RUN #3: LONG RUN

Complete a 15- to 20-mile run @ 9:23/mile pace (24K to 32K run @ 5:49/kilometer pace)

3:55 Boston Marathon Training Plan

RI = Rest Interval; which may be a timed rest/recovery interval or a distance that you walk/jog. Key Run #1 always begins with a 10- to 20 minute warmup and ends with a 10-minute cooldown Metric workout equivalents appear in bold italics.

WEEK	KEY RUN #1	KEY RUN #2	KEY RUN #3
16	3 × 1600 in 7:30 (400 RI)	2 miles *(3K)* easy 2 miles at 8:04 *(3K at 5:00)* 2 miles *(3K)* easy	13 miles at 9:27 *(21K at 5:53)*
15	4 × 800 in 3:37 (2 min RI)	1 mile *(1.5K)* easy 5 miles at 8:57 *(8K at 5:34)* 1 mile *(1.5K)* easy	15 miles at 9:42 *(24K at 6:02)*
14	1200 in 5:32 (200 RI); 1000 in 4:34 (200 RI); 800 in 3:37 (200 RI); 600 in 2:42 (200 RI); 400 in 1:47 (200 RI)	1 mile *(1.5K)* easy 5 miles at 8:34 *(8K at 5:19)* 1 mile *(1.5K)* easy	17 miles at 9:42 *(27K at 6:02)*
13	5 × 1000 in 4:34 (400 RI)	1 mile *(1.5K)* easy 4 miles at 8:19 *(6.5K at 5:10)* 1 mile *(1.5K)* easy	20 miles at 9:57 *(32K at 6:11)*
12	3 × 1600 in 7:30 (400 RI)	2 miles *(3K)* easy 3 miles at 8:04 *(5K at 5:00)* 1 mile *(1.5K)* easy	18 miles at 9:42 *(29K at 6:02)*
11	2 × 1200 in 5:32 (2 min RI); 4 × 800 in 3:37 (2 min RI)	1 mile *(1.5K)* easy 5 miles at 8:19 *(8K at 5:10)* 1 mile *(1.5K)* easy	20 miles at 9:42 *(32K at 6:02)*
10	6 × 800 in 3:37 (90 sec RI)	1 mile *(1.5K)* easy 6 miles at 8:34 *(10K at 5:19)* 1 mile *(1.5K)* easy	13 miles at 9:12 *(21K at 5:43)*
9	2 × (6 × 400 in 1:47) (90 sec RI (2 min 30 sec RI between sets)	2 miles *(3K)* easy 3 miles at 8:04 *(5K at 5:00)* 1 mile *(1.5K)* easy	18 miles at 9:27 *(29K at 5:53)*
8	2 × 1600 in 7:30 (60 sec RI) 2 × 800 in 3:37 (60 sec RI)	1 mile *(1.5K)* easy 4 miles at 8:19 *(6.5K at 5:10)* 1 mile *(1.5K)* easy	20 miles at 9:27 *(32K at 5:53)*
7	3 × (2 × 1200 in 5:32) (2 min RI) (4 min RI between sets)	10 min warmup 10 miles at 8:57 *(16K at 5:34)* 10 min cooldown	15 miles at 9:17 *(24K at 5:46)*
6	1000 in 4:34; 2000 in 9:28; 1000 in 4:34; 1000 in 4:34 (400 RI)	1 mile *(1.5K)* easy 5 miles at 8:57 *(8K at 5:34)* 1 mile *(1.5K)* easy	20 miles at 9:27 *(32K at 5:53)*

WEEK	KEY RUN #1	KEY RUN #2	KEY RUN #3
5	3 × 1600 in 7:30 (400 RI)	10 min warmup 10 miles at 8:57 *(16K at 5:34)* 10 min cooldown	15 miles at 9:12 *(24K at 5:43)*
4	10 × 400 in 1:47 (400 RI)	10 min warmup 8 miles at 8:57 *(13K at 5:34)* 10 min cooldown	20 miles at 9:12 *(32K at 5:43)*
3	8 × 800 in 3:37 (90 sec RI)	1 mile *(1.5K)* easy 5 miles at 8:19 *(8K at 5:10)* 1 mile *(1.5K)* easy	13 miles at 8:57 *(21K at 5:34)*
2	5 × 1000 in 4:34 (400RI)	2 miles *(3K)* easy 3 miles at 8:04 *(5K at 5:00)* 1 mile *(1.5K)* easy	10 miles at 8:57 *(16K at 5:34)*
1	6 × 400 in 1:47 (400 RI)	10 min warmup 3 miles at 8:57 *(5K at 5:34)* 10 min cooldown	MARATHON 26.2 miles at 8:57 *(42.2K at 5:34)*

BQ for Women 50 to 54: 4:00

Qualifying for Boston is realistic if you can:

Run a 5K in 24:40; a 10K in 51:36; a half-marathon in 1:54:20.

If you can complete one of each of the **three** key runs in the **same** week:

KEY RUN #1: TRACK REPEATS
(complete one of the workouts listed below)

6 × 800 @ 3:42 with 400 recovery jog between repeats

5 × 1000 @ 4:40 with 400 recovery jog between repeats

4 × 1200M @ 5:39 with 400 recovery jog between repeats

3 × 1600 @ 7:40 with 400 recovery jog between repeats

KEY RUN #2: TEMPO RUN
(complete one of the tempo runs)

After a 1-mile warmup, complete a 3-mile run in 24:39 (1.5K warmup; 5K run in 25:30)

After a 1-mile warmup, complete a 5-mile run in 42:20 (1.5K warmup; 8K run in 42:08)

After a 1-mile warmup, complete an 8-mile training run in 69:34 (1.5K warmup; 13K run in 70:25)

KEY RUN #3: LONG RUN

Complete a 15- to 20-mile run @ 9:34/mile pace (24K to 32K @ 5:56/kilometer pace)

4:00 Boston Marathon Training Plan

RI = Rest Interval; which may be a timed rest/recovery interval or a distance that you walk/jog.
Key Run #1 always begins with a 10- to 20-minute warmup and ends with a 10-minute cooldown

Metric workout equivalents appear in bold italics.

WEEK	KEY RUN #1	KEY RUN #2	KEY RUN #3
16	3 × 1600 in 7:40 (400 RI)	2 miles *(3K)* easy 2 miles at 8:13 *(3K at 5:06)* 2 miles *(3K)* easy	13 miles at 9:39 *(21K at 6:00)*
15	4 × 800 in 3:42 (2 min RI)	1 mile *(1.5K)* easy 5 miles at 9:09 *(8K at 5:41)* 1 mile *(1.5K)* easy	15 miles at 9:54 *(24K at 6:09)*
14	1200 in 5:39 (200 RI); 1000 in 4:40 (200 RI); 800 in 3:42 (200 RI); 600 in 2:45 (200 RI); 400 in 1:49 (200 RI)	1 mile *(1.5K)* easy 5 miles at 8:43 *(8K at 5:25)* 1 mile *(1.5K)* easy	17 miles at 9:54 *(27K at 6:09)*
13	5 × 1000 in 4:40 (400 RI)	1 mile *(1.5K)* easy 4 miles at 8:28 *(6.5K at 5:16)* 1 mile *(1.5K)* easy	20 miles at 10:09 *(32K at 6:18)*
12	3 × 1600 in 7:40 (400 RI)	2 miles *(3K)* easy 3 miles at 8:13 *(5K at 5:06)* 1 mile *(1.5K)* easy	18 miles at 9:54 *(29K at 6:09)*
11	2 × 1200 in 5:39 (2 min RI); 4 × 800 in 3:42 (2 min RI)	1 mile *(1.5K)* easy 5 miles at 8:28 *(8K at 5:16)* 1 mile *(1.5K)* easy	20 miles at 9:54 *(32K at 6:09)*
10	6 × 800 in 3:42 (90 sec RI)	1 mile *(1.5K)* easy 6 miles at 8:43 *(10K at 5:25)* 1 mile *(1.5K)* easy	13 miles at 9:24 *(21K at 5:50)*
9	2 × (6 × 400 in 1:49) (90 sec RI) (2 min 30 sec RI between sets)	2 miles *(3K)* easy 3 miles at 8:13 *(5K at 5:06)* 1 mile *(1.5K)* easy	18 miles at 9:39 *(29K at 6:00)*
8	2 × 1600 in 7:40 (60 sec RI); 2 × 800 in 3:42 (60 sec RI)	1 mile *(1.5K)* easy 4 miles at 8:28 *(6.5K at 5:16)* 1 mile *(1.5K)* easy	20 miles at 9:39 *(32K at 6:00)*
7	3 × (2 × 1200 in 5:39) (2 min RI) (4 min RI between sets)	10 min warmup 10 miles at 9:09 *(16K at 5:41)* 10 min cooldown	15 miles at 9:29 *(24K at 5:53)*

WEEK	KEY RUN #1	KEY RUN #2	KEY RUN #3
6	1000 in 4:40; 2000 in 9:40; 1000 in 4:40; 1000 in 4:40 (400 RI)	1 mile *(1.5K)* easy 5 miles at 9:09 *(8K at 5:41)* 1 mile *(1.5K)* easy	20 miles at 9:39 *(32K at 6:00)*
5	3 × 1600 in 7:40 (400 RI)	10 min warmup 10 miles at 9:09 *(16K at 5:41)* 10 min cooldown	15 miles at 9:24 *(24K at 5:50)*
4	10 × 400 in 1:49 (400 RI)	10 min warmup 8 miles at 9:09 *(13K at 5:41)* 10 min cooldown	20 miles at 9:24 *(32K at 5:50)*
3	8 × 800 in 3:42 (90 sec RI)	1 mile *(1.5K)* easy 5 miles at 8:28 *(8K at 5:16)* 1 mile *(1.5K)* easy	13 miles at 9:09 *(21K at 5:41)*
2	5 × 1000 in 4:40 (400 RI)	2 miles *(3K)* easy 3 miles at 8:13 *(5K at 5:06)* 1 mile *(1.5K)* easy	10 miles at 9:09 *(16K at 5:41)*
1	6 × 400 in 1:49 (400 RI)	10 min warmup 3 miles at 9:09 *(5K at 5:41)* 10 min cooldown	MARATHON 26.2 miles at 9:09 *(42.2K at 5:41)*

BQ for Men 65 to 69 and Women 55 to 59: 4:10

Qualifying for Boston is realistic if you can:

Run a 5K in 25:40; a 10K in 53:45; a half-marathon in 1:59:00.

If you can complete one of each of the **three** key runs in the same week:

KEY RUN #1: TRACK REPEATS
(complete one of the workouts listed below)

6 × 800 @ 3:52 with 400 recovery jog between repeats

5 × 1000 @ 4:52 with 400 recovery jog between repeats

4 × 1200 @ 5:54 with 400 recovery jog between repeats

3 × 1600 @ 8:00 with 400 recovery jog between repeats

KEY RUN #2: TEMPO RUN
(complete one of the tempo runs)

After a 1-mile warmup, complete a 3-mile run in 25:39 (1.5K warmup; 5K run in 26:30)

After a 1-mile warmup, complete a 5-mile run in 44:00 (1.5K warmup; 8K run in 43:44)

After a 1-mile warmup, complete an 8-mile run in 72:24 (1.5K warmup; 13K run in 71:01)

KEY RUN #3: LONG RUN

Complete a 15- to 20-mile run @ 9:57/mile pace (24K to 32K run @ 6:10/kilometer pace)

4:10 Boston Marathon Training Plan

RI = Rest Interval; which may be a timed rest/recovery interval or a distance that you walk/jog.
Key Run #1 always begins with a 10- to 20-minute warmup and ends with a 10-minute cooldown.
Metric workout equivalents appear in bold italics.

WEEK	KEY RUN #1	KEY RUN #2	KEY RUN #3
16	3 × 1600 in 8:00 (400 RI)	2 miles *(3K)* easy 2 miles at 8:33 *(3K at 5:18)* 2 miles *(3K)* easy	13 miles at 10:02 *(21K at 6:14)*
15	4 × 800 in 3:52 (2 min RI)	1 mile *(1.5K)* easy 5 miles at 9:32 *(8K at 5:55)* 1 mile *(1.5K)* easy	15 miles at 10:17 *(24K at 6:23)*
14	1200 in 5:54 (200 RI); 1000 in 4:52 (200 RI); 800 in 3:52 (200 RI); 600 in 2:53 (200 RI); 400 in 1:54 (200 RI)	1 mile *(1.5K)* easy 5 miles at 9:03 *(8K at 5:37)* 1 mile *(1.5K)* easy	17 miles at 10:17 *(27K at 6:23)*
13	5 × 1000 in 4:52 (400 RI)	1 mile *(1.5K)* easy 4 miles at 8:48 *(6.5K at 5:28)* 1 mile *(1.5K)* easy	20 miles at 10:32 *(32K at 6:32)*
12	3 × 1600 in 8:00 (400 RI)	2 miles *(3K)* easy 3 miles at 8:33 *(5K at 5:18)* 1 mile *(1.5K)* easy	18 miles at 10:17 *(29K at 6:23)*
11	2 × 1200 in 5:54 (2 min RI); 4 × 800 in 3:52 (2 min RI)	1 mile *(1.5K)* easy 5 miles at 8:48 *(8K at 5:28)* 1 mile *(1.5K)* easy	20 miles at 10:17 *(32K at 6:23)*
10	6 × 800 in 3:52 (90 sec RI)	1 mile *(1.5K)* easy 6 miles at 9:03 *(10K at 5:37)* 1 mile *(1.5K)* easy	13 miles at 9:47 *(21K at 6:04)*
9	2 × (6 × 400 in 1:54) (90 sec RI) (2 min 30 sec RI between sets)	2 miles *(3K)* easy 3 miles at 8:33 *(5K at 5:18)* 1 mile *(1.5K)* easy	18 miles at 10:02 *(29K at 6:14)*
8	2 × 1600 in 8:00 (60 sec RI); 2 × 800 in 3:52 (60 sec RI)	1 mile *(1.5K)* easy 4 miles at 8:48 *(6.5K at 5:28)* 1 mile *(1.5K)* easy	20 miles at 10:02 *(32K at 6:14)*
7	3 × (2 × 1200 in 5:54) (2 min RI) (4 min RI between sets)	10 min warmup 10 miles at 9:03 *(16K at 5:55)* 10 min cooldown	15 miles at 9:52 *(24K at 6:07)*
6	1000 in 4:52; 2000 in 10:05; 1000 in 4:52; 1000 in 4:52 (400 RI)	1 mile *(1.5K)* easy 5 miles at 9:03 *(8K at 5:55)* 1 mile *(1.5K)* easy	20 miles at 10:02 *(32K at 6:14)*

WEEK	KEY RUN #1	KEY RUN #2	KEY RUN #3
5	3 × 1600 in 8:00 (400 RI)	10 min warmup 10 miles at 9:03 *(16K at 5:55)* 10 min cooldown	15 miles at 9:47 *(24K at 6:04)*
4	10 × 400 in 1:54 (400 RI)	10 min warmup 0 miles at 9.03 *(13K at 5:55)* 10 min cooldown	20 miles at 9:47 *(32K at 6:04)*
3	8 × 800 in 3:52 (90 sec RI)	1 mile *(1.5K)* easy 5 miles at 8:48 *(8K at 5:28)* 1 mile *(1.5K)* easy	13 miles at 9:32 *(21K at 5:55)*
2	5 × 1000 in 4:52 (400 RI)	2 miles *(3K)* easy 3 miles at 8:33 *(5K at 5:18)* 1 mile *(1.5K)* easy	10 miles at 9:32 *(16K at 5:55)*
1	6 × 400 in 1:54 (400 RI)	10 min warmup 3 miles at 9:32 *(5K at 5:55)* 10 min cooldown	MARATHON 26.2 miles at 9:32 *(42.2K at 5:55)*

BQ for Men 70 to 74 and Women 60 to 64: 4:25

Qualifying for Boston is realistic if you can:

Run a 5K in 27:15; a 10K in 57:00; a half-marathon in 2:06:20.

If you can complete one of each of the **three** key runs in the **same** week:

KEY RUN #1: TRACK REPEATS
(complete one of the workouts listed below)

6 × 800 @ 4:07 with 400 recovery jog between repeats

5 × 1000 @ 5:11 with 400 recovery jog between repeats

4 × 1200 @ 6:17 with 400 recovery jog between repeats

3 × 1600 @ 8:30 with 400 recovery jog between repeats

KEY RUN #2: TEMPO RUN
(complete one of the tempo runs)

After a 1-mile warmup, complete a 3-mile run in 27:09 (1.5K warmup; 5K run in 28:05)

After a 1-mile warmup, complete a 5-mile run in 46:40 (1.5K warmup; 8K run in 46:16)

After a 1-mile warmup, complete an 8-mile run in 76:40 (1.5K warmup; 13K run in 77:08)

KEY RUN #3: LONG RUN

Complete a 15- to 20-mile run @ 10:32/mile pace (24K to 32K run @ 6:32/kilometer pace)

4:25 Boston Marathon Training Plan

RI = Rest Interval; which may be a timed rest/recovery interval or a distance that you walk/jog.
Key Run #1 always begins with a 10- to 20-minute warmup and ends with a 10-minute cooldown.
Metric workout equivalents appear in bold italics.

WEEK	KEY RUN #1	KEY RUN #2	KEY RUN #3
16	3 × 1600 in 8:30 (400 RI)	2 miles *(3K)* easy 2 miles at 9:03 *(3K at 5:37)* 2 miles *(3K)* easy	13 miles at 10:36 *(21K at 6:36)*
15	4 × 800 in 4:07 (2 min RI)	1 mile *(1.5K)* easy 5 miles at 10:06 *(8K at 6:17)* 1 mile *(1.5K)* easy	15 miles at 10:51 *(24K at 6:45)*
14	1200 in 6:17 (200 RI); 1000 in 5:11 (200 RI); 800 in 4:07 (200 RI); 600 in 3:04 (200 RI); 400 in 2:02 (200 RI)	1 mile *(1.5K)* easy 5 miles at 9:33 *(8K at 5:56)* 1 mile *(1.5K)* easy	17 miles at 10:51 *(27K at 6:45)*
13	5 × 1000 in 5:11 (400 RI)	1 mile *(1.5K)* easy 4 miles at 9:18 *(6.5K at 5:47)* 1 mile *(1.5K)* easy	20 miles at 11:06 *(32K at 6:54)*
12	3 × 1600 in 8:30 (400 RI)	2 miles *(3K)* easy 3 miles at 9:03 *(5K at 5:37)* 1 mile *(1.5K)* easy	18 miles at 10:51 *(29K at 6:45)*
11	2 × 1200 in 6:17 (2 min RI); 4 × 800 in 4:07 (2 min RI)	1 mile *(1.5K)* easy 5 miles at 9:18 *(8K at 5:47)* 1 mile *(1.5K)* easy	20 miles at 10:51 *(32K at 6:45)*
10	6 × 800 in 4:07 (90 sec RI)	1 mile *(1.5K)* easy 6 miles at 9:33 *(10K at 5:56)* 1 mile *(1.5K)* easy	13 miles at 10:21 *(21K at 6:26)*
9	2 × (6 × 400 in 2:02) (90 sec RI) (2 min 30 sec RI between sets)	2 miles *(3K)* easy 3 miles at 9:03 *(5K at 5:37)* 1 mile *(1.5K)* easy	18 miles at 10:36 *(29K at 6:36)*
8	2 × 1600 in 8:30 (60 sec RI); 2 × 800 in 4:07 (60 sec RI)	1 mile *(1.5K)* easy 4 miles at 9:18 *(6.5K at 5:47)* 1 mile *(1.5K)* easy	20 miles at 10:36 *(32K at 6:36)*
7	3 × (2 × 1200 in 6:17) (2 min RI) (4 min RI between sets)	10 min warmup 10 miles at 10:06 *(16K at 6:17)* 10 min cooldown	15 miles at 10:26 *(24K at 6:29)*
6	1000 in 5:11; 2000 in 10:43; 1000 in 5:11; 1000 in 5:11 (400 RI)	1 mile *(1.5K)* easy 5 miles at 10:06 *(8K at 6:17)* 1 mile *(1.5K)* easy	20 miles at 10:36 *(32K at 6:36)*

WEEK	KEY RUN #1	KEY RUN #2	KEY RUN #3
5	3 × 1600 in 8:30 (400 RI)	10 min warmup 10 miles at 10:06 *(16K at 6:17)* 10 min cooldown	15 miles at 10:21 *(24K at 6:26)*
4	10 × 400 in 2:02 (400 RI)	10 min warmup 8 miles at 10:06 *(13K at 6:17)* 10 min cooldown	20 miles at 10:21 *(32K at 6:26)*
3	8 × 800 in 4:07 (90 sec RI)	1 mile *(1.5K)* easy 5 miles at 9:18 *(8K at 5:47)* 1 mile *(1.5K)* easy	13 miles at 10:06 *(21K at 6:17)*
2	5 × 1000 in 5:11 (400 RI)	2 miles *(3K)* easy 3 miles at 9:03 *(5K at 5:37)* 1 mile *(1.5K)* easy	10 miles at 10:06 *(16K at 6:17)*
1	6 × 400 in 2:02 (400 RI)	10 minute warmup 3 miles at 10:06 *(5K at 6:17)* 10 min cooldown	MARATHON 26.2 miles at 10:06 *(42.2K at 6:17)*

BQ for Men 75 to 79 and Women 65 to 69: 4:40

Qualifying for Boston is realistic if you can:

Run a 5K in 28:45; a 10K in 60:05; a half-marathon in 2:13:15.

If you can complete one of each of the **three** key runs in the same week:

KEY RUN #1: TRACK REPEATS
(complete one of the workouts listed below)

6 × 800 @ 4:22 with 400 recovery jog between repeats

5 × 1000 @ 5:29 with 400 recovery jog between repeats

4 × 1200 @ 6:38 with 400 recovery jog between repeats

3 × 1600 @ 8:59 with 400 recovery jog between repeats

KEY RUN #2: TEMPO RUN
(complete one of the tempo runs)

After a 1-mile warmup, complete a 3-mile run in 28:36 (1.5K warmup; 5K run in 29:35)

After a 1-mile warmup, complete a 5-mile run in 48:55 (1.5K warmup; 8K run in 48:40)

After a 1-mile warmup, complete an 8-mile run in 80:32 (1.5K warmup; 13K run in 81:02)

KEY RUN #3: LONG RUN

Complete a 15- to 20-mile run @ 11:05/mile pace (24K to 32K run @ 6:53/kilometer pace)

4:40 Boston Marathon Training Plan

RI = Rest Interval; which may be a timed rest/recovery interval or a distance that you walk/jog. Key Run #1 always begins with a 10- to 20-minute warmup and ends with a 10-minute cooldown.

Metric workout equivalents appear in bold italics.

WEEK	KEY RUN #1	KEY RUN #2	KEY RUN #3
16	3 × 1600 in 8:59 (400 RI)	2 miles *(3K)* easy 2 miles at 9:32 *(3K at 5:55)* 2 miles *(3K)* easy	13 miles at 11:10 *(21K at 6:57)*
15	4 × 800 in 4:22 (2 min RI)	1 mile *(1.5K)* easy 5 miles at 10:40 *(8K at 6:38)* 1 mile *(1.5K)* easy	15 miles at 11:25 *(24K at 7:06)*
14	1200 in 6:38 (200 RI); 1000 in 5:29 (200 RI); 800 in 4:22 (200 RI); 600 in 3:15 (200 RI); 400 in 2:09 (200 RI)	1 mile *(1.5K)* easy 5 miles at 10:02 *(8K at 6:14)* 1 mile *(1.5K)* easy	17 miles at 11:25 *(27K at 7:06)*
13	5 × 1000 in 5:29 (400 RI)	1 mile *(1.5K)* easy 4 miles at 9:47 *(6.5K at 6:05)* 1 mile *(1.5K)* easy	20 miles at 11:40 *(32K at 7:15)*
12	3 × 1600 in 8:59 (400 RI)	2 miles *(3K)* easy 3 miles at 9:32 *(5K at 5:55)* 1 mile *(1.5K)* easy	18 miles at 11:25 *(29K at 7:06)*
11	2 × 1200 in 6:38 (2 min RI); 4 × 800 in 4:22 (2 min RI)	1 mile *(1.5K)* easy 5 miles at 9:47 *(8K at 6:05)* 1 mile *(1.5K)* easy	20 miles at 11:25 *(32K at 7:06)*
10	6 × 800 in 4:22 (90 sec RI)	1 mile *(1.5K)* easy 6 miles at 10:02 *(10K at 6:14)* 1 mile *(1.5K)* easy	13 miles at 10:55 *(21K at 6:47)*
9	2 × (6 × 400 in 2:09) (90 sec RI) (2 min 30 sec RI between sets)	2 miles *(3K)* easy 3 miles at 9:32 *(5K at 5:55)* 1 mile *(1.5K)* easy	18 miles at 11:10 *(29K at 6:57)*
8	2 × 1600 in 8:59 (60 sec RI) 2 × 800 in 4:22 (60 sec RI)	1 mile *(1.5K)* easy 4 miles at 9:47 *(6.5K at 6:05)* 1 mile *(1.5K)* easy	20 miles at 11:10 *(32K at 6:57)*
7	3 × (2 × 1200 in 6:38) (2 min RI) (4 min RI between sets)	10 min warmup 10 miles at 10:40 *(16K at 6:38)* 10 min cooldown	15 miles at 11:00 *(24K at 6:50)*
6	1000 in 5:29; 2000 in 11:19; 1000 in 5:29; 1000 in 5:29 (400 RI)	1 mile *(1.5K)* easy 5 miles at 10:40 *(8K at 6:38)* 1 mile *(1.5K)* easy	20 miles at 11:10 *(32K at 6:57)*

WEEK	KEY RUN #1	KEY RUN #2	KEY RUN #3
5	3 × 1600 in 8:59 (400 RI)	10 min warmup 10 miles at 10:40 *(16K at 6:38)* 10 min cooldown	15 miles at 10:55 *(24K at 6:47)*
4	10 × 400 in 2:09 (400 RI)	10 min warmup 8 miles at 10:40 *(13K at 6:38)* 10 min cooldown	20 miles at 10:55 *(32K at 6:47)*
3	8 × 800 in 4:22 (90 sec RI)	1 mile *(1.5K)* easy 5 miles at 9:47 *(8K at 6:05)* 1 mile *(1.5K)* easy	13 miles at 10:40 *(21K at 6:38)*
2	5 × 1000 in 5:29 (400 RI)	2 miles *(3K)* easy 3 miles at 9:32 *(5K at 5:55)* 1 mile *(1.5K)* easy	10 miles at 10:40 *(16K at 6:38)*
1	6 × 400 in 2:09 (400 RI)	10 min warmup 3 miles at 10:40 *(5K at 6:38)* 10 min cooldown	MARATHON 26.2 miles at 10:40 *(42.2K at 6:38)*

BQ for Men 80 and over and Women 70 to 74: 4:55

Qualifying for Boston is realistic if you can:

Run a 5K in 30:20; a 10K in 63:28; a half-marathon in 2:20:36.

If you can complete one of each of the **three** key runs in the **same** week:

KEY RUN #1: TRACK REPEATS
(complete one of the workouts listed below)

6 × 800 @ 4:37 with 400 recovery jog between repeats

5 × 1000 @ 5:48 with 400 recovery jog between repeats

4 × 1200 @ 7:00 with 400 recovery jog between repeats

3 × 1600 @ 9:29 with a 400 recovery jog between repeats

KEY RUN #2: TEMPO RUN
(complete one of the tempo runs)

After a 1-mile warmup, complete a 3-mile run in 30:09 (1.5K warmup; 5K run in 31:20)

After a 1-mile warmup, complete a 5-mile run in 51:30 (1.5K warmup; 8K run in 51:12)

After a 1-mile warmup, complete an 8-mile run in 84:24 (1.5K warmup; 13K run in 85:09)

KEY RUN #3: LONG RUN

Complete a 15- to 20-mile run @ 11:40/mile pace (24K to 32K run @ 7:15/kilometer pace)

4:55 Boston Marathon Training Plan

RI = Rest Interval; which may be a timed rest/recovery interval or a distance that you walk/jog.
Key Run #1 always begins with a 10- to 20-minute warmup and ends with a 10-minute
cooldown.
Metric workout equivalents appear in bold italics.

WEEK	KEY RUN #1	KEY RUN #2	KEY RUN #3
16	3 × 1600 in 9:29 (400 RI)	2 miles (*3K*) easy 2 miles at 10:03 (*3K at 6:14*) 2 miles (*3K*) easy	13 miles at 11:45 (*21K at 7:19*)
15	4 × 800 in 4:37 (2 min RI)	1 mile (*1.5K*) easy 5 miles at 11:15 (*8K at 7:00*) 1 mile (*1.5K*) easy	15 miles at 12:00 (*24K at 7:28*)
14	1200 in 7:01 (200 RI); 1000 in 5:48 (200 RI); 800 in 4:37 (200 RI); 600 in 3:27 (200 RI); 400 in 2:16 (200 RI)	1 mile (*1.5K*) easy 5 miles at 10:33 (*8K at 6:33*) 1 mile (*1.5K*) easy	17 miles at 12:00 (*27K at 7:28*)
13	5 × 1000 in 5:48 (400 RI)	1 mile (*1.5K*) easy 4 miles at 10:18 (*6.5K at 6:24*) 1 mile (*1.5K*) easy	20 miles at 12:15 (*32K at 7:37*)
12	3 × 1600 in 9:29 (400 RI)	2 miles (*3K*) easy 3 miles at 10:03 (*5K at 6:14*) 1 mile (*1.5K*) easy	18 miles at 12:00 (*29K at 7:28*)
11	2 × 1200 in 7:01 (2 min RI); 4 × 800 in 4:37 (2 min RI)	1 mile (*1.5K*) easy 5 miles at 10:18 (*8K at 6:24*) 1 mile (*1.5K*) easy	20 miles at 12:00 (*32K at 7:28*)
10	6 × 800 in 4:37 (90 sec RI)	1 mile (*1.5K*) easy 6 miles at 10:33 (*10K at 6:33*) 1 mile (*1.5K*) easy	13 miles at 11:30 (*21K at 7:09*)
9	2 × (6 × 400 in 2:16) (90 sec RI) (2 min 30 sec RI between sets)	2 miles (*3K*) easy 3 miles at 10:03 (*5K at 6:14*) 1 mile (*1.5K*) easy	18 miles at 11:45 (*29K at 7:19*)
8	2 × 1600 in 9:29 (60 sec RI) 2 × 800 in 4:37 (60 sec RI)	1 mile (*1.5K*) easy 4 miles at 10:18 (*6.5K at 6:24*) 1 mile (*1.5K*) easy	20 miles at 11:45 (*32K at 7:19*)
7	3 × (2 × 1200 in 7:01) (2 min RI) (4 min RI between sets)	10 min warmup 10 miles at 11:15 (*16K at 7:00*) 10 min cooldown	15 miles at 11:35 (*24K at 7:12*)
6	1000 in 5:48; 2000 in 11:57; 1000 in 5:48; 1000 in 5:48 (400 RI)	1 mile (*1.5K*) easy 5 miles at 11:15 (*8K at 7:00*) 1 mile (*1.5K*) easy	20 miles at 11:45 (*32K at 7:19*)

WEEK	KEY RUN #1	KEY RUN #2	KEY RUN #3
5	3 × 1600 in 9:29 (400 RI)	10 min warmup 10 miles at 11:15 *(16K at 7:00)* 10 min cooldown	15 miles at 11:30 *(24K at 7:09)*
4	10 × 400 in 2:16 (400 RI)	10 min warmup 8 miles at 11:15 *(13K at 7:00)* 10 min cooldown	20 miles at 11:30 *(32K at 7:09)*
3	8 × 800 in 4:37 (90 sec RI)	1 mile *(1.5K)* easy 5 miles at 10:18 *(8K at 6:24)* 1 mile *(1.5K)* easy	13 miles at 11:15 *(21K at 7:00)*
2	5 × 1000 in 5:48 (400 RI)	2 miles *(3K)* easy 3 miles at 10:03 *(5K at 6:14)* 1 mile *(1.5K)* easy	10 miles at 11:15 *(16K at 7:00)*
1	6 × 400 in 2:16 (400 RI)	10 min warmup 3 miles at 11:15 *(5K at 7:00)* 10 min cooldown	MARATHON 26.2 miles at 11:15 *(42.2K at 7:00)*

BQ for Women 75 to 79: 5:10

Qualifying for Boston is realistic if you can:

Run a 5K in 31:50; a 10K in 1:06:30; a half-marathon in 2:27:30.

If you can complete one of each of the **three** key runs in the same week:

KEY RUN #1: TRACK REPEATS
(complete one of the workouts listed below)

6 × 800 @ 4:52 with 400 recovery jog between repeats

5 × 1000 @ 6:05 with 400 recovery jog between repeats

4 × 1200 @ 7:23 with 400 recovery jog between repeats

3 × 1600 @ 9:58 with 400M recovery jog between repeats

KEY RUN #2: TEMPO RUN
(complete one of the tempo runs)

After a 1-mile warmup, complete a 3-mile run in 31:36 (1.5K warmup; 5K run in 32:40)

After a 1-mile warmup, complete a 5-mile run in 54:00 (1.5K warmup; 8K run in 53:32)

After a 1-mile warmup, complete an 8-mile run in 88:00 (1.5K warmup; 13K run in 89:03)

KEY RUN #3: LONG RUN

Complete a 15- to 20-mile run @ 12:15/mile pace (24K to 32K @ 7:37/kilometer pace)

5:10 Boston Marathon Training Plan

RI = Rest Interval; which may be a timed rest/recovery interval or a distance that you walk/jog. Key Run #1 always begins with a 10- to 20-minute warmup and ends with a 10-minute cooldown.

Metric workout equivalents appear in bold italics.

WEEK	KEY RUN #1	KEY RUN #2	KEY RUN #3
16	3 × 1600 in 9:58 (400 RI)	2 miles *(3K)* easy 2 miles at 10:32 *(3K at 6:32)* 2 miles *(3K)* easy	13 miles at 12:19 *(21K at 7:39)*
15	4 × 800 in 4:52 (2 min RI)	1 mile *(1.5K)* easy 5 miles at 11:49 *(8K at 7:20)* 1 mile *(1.5K)* easy	15 miles at 12:34 *(24K at 7:48)*
14	1200 in 7:23 (200 RI); 1000 in 6:06 (200 RI); 800 in 4:52 (200 RI); 600 in 3:38 (200 RI); 400 in 2:23 (200 RI)	1 mile *(1.5K)* easy 5 miles at 11:02 *(8K at 6:51)* 1 mile *(1.5K)* easy	17 miles at 12:34 *(27K at 7:48)*
13	5 × 1000 in 6:06 (400 RI)	1 mile *(1.5K)* easy 4 miles at 10:47 *(6.5K at 6:42)* 1 mile *(1.5K)* easy	20 miles at 12:49 *(32K at 7:57)*
12	3 × 1600 in 9:58 (400 RI)	2 miles *(3K)* easy 3 miles at 10:32 *(5K at 6:32)* 1 mile *(1.5K)* easy	18 miles at 12:34 *(29K at 7:48)*
11	2 × 1200 in 7:23 (2 min RI); 4 × 800 in 4:52 (2 min RI)	1 mile *(1.5K)* easy 5 miles at 10:47 *(8K at 6:42)* 1 mile *(1.5K)* easy	20 miles at 12:34 *(32K at 7:48)*
10	6 × 800 in 4:52 (90 sec RI)	1 mile *(1.5K)* easy 6 miles at 11:02 *(10K at 6:51)* 1 mile *(1.5K)* easy	13 miles at 12:04 *(21K at 7:29)*
9	2 × (6 × 400 in 2:23) (90 sec RI) (2 min 30 sec RI between sets)	2 miles *(3K)* easy 3 miles at 10:32 *(5K at 6:32)* 1 mile *(1.5K)* easy	18 miles at 12:19 *(29K at 7:39)*
8	2 × 1600 in 9:58 (60 sec RI); 2 × 800 in 4:52 (60 sec RI)	1 mile *(1.5K)* easy 4 miles at 10:47 *(6.5K at 6:42)* 1 mile *(1.5K)* easy	20 miles at 12:19 *(32K at 7:39)*
7	3 × (2 × 1200 in 7:23) (2 min RI) (4 min RI between sets)	10 min warmup 10 miles at 11:49 *(16K at 7:20)* 10 min cooldown	15 miles at 12:09 *(24K at 7:32)*
6	1000 in 6:06; 2000 in 12:33; 1000 in 6:06; 1000 in 6:06 (400 RI)	1 mile *(1.5K)* easy 5 miles at 11:49 *(8K at 7:20)* 1 mile *(1.5K)* easy	20 miles at 12:19 *(32K at 7:39)*

WEEK	KEY RUN #1	KEY RUN #2	KEY RUN #3
5	3 × 1600 in 9:58 (400 RI)	10 min warmup 10 miles at 11:49 *(16K at 7:20)* 10 min cooldown	15 miles at 12:04 *(24K at 7:29)*
4	10 × 400 in 2:23 (400 RI)	10 min warmup 8 miles at 11:49 *(13K at 7:20)* 10 min cooldown	20 miles at 12:04 *(32K at 7:29)*
3	8 × 800 in 4:52 (90 sec RI)	1 mile *(1.5K)* easy 5 miles at 10:47 *(8K at 6:42)* 1 mile *(1.5K)* easy	13 miles at 11:49 *(21K at 7:20)*
2	5 × 1000 in 6:06 (400 RI)	2 miles *(3K)* easy 3 miles at 10:32 *(5K at 6:32)* 1 mile *(1.5K)* easy	10 miles at 11:49 *(16K at 7:20)*
1	6 × 400 in 2:23 (400 RI)	10 min warmup 3 miles at 11:49 *(5K at 7:20)* 10 min cooldown	MARATHON 26.2 miles at 11:49 *(42.2K at 7:20)*

BQ for Women 80 and over: 5:25

Qualifying for Boston is realistic if you can:

Run a 5K in 33:25; a 10K in 71:00; a half-marathon in 2:34:30.

If you can complete one of each of the **three** key runs in the **same** week:

KEY RUN #1: TRACK REPEATS
(complete one of the workouts listed below)

6 × 800 @ 5:06 with 400 recovery jog between repeats

5 × 1000 @ 6:25 with 400 recovery jog between repeats

4 × 1200 @ 7:46 with 400 recovery jog between repeats

3 × 1600 @ 10:30 with 400 recovery jog between repeats

KEY RUN #2: TEMPO RUN
(complete one of the tempo runs)

After a 1-mile warmup, complete a 3-mile run in 33:12 (1.5K warmup; 5K run in 34:18)

After a 1-mile warmup, complete a 5-mile run in 56:40 (1.5K warmup; 8K run in 56:08)

After a 1-mile warmup, complete an 8-mile run in 92:00 (1.5K warmup, 13K run in 93:10)

KEY RUN #3: LONG RUN

Complete a 15- to 20-mile run @ 12:45/mile pace (24K to 32K run @ 7:57/kilometer pace)

5:25 Boston Marathon Training Plan

RI = Rest Interval; which may be a timed rest/recovery interval or a distance that you walk/jog.
Key Run #1 always begins with a 10- to 20-minute warmup and ends with a 10-minute cooldown.
Metric workout equivalents appear in bold italics.

WEEK	KEY RUN #1	KEY RUN #2	KEY RUN #3
16	3 × 1600 in 10:30 (400 RI)	2 miles (3K) easy 2 miles at 11:02 (3K at 6:51) 2 miles (3K) easy	13 miles at 12:53 (21K at 8:01)
15	4 × 800 in 5:06 (2 min RI)	1 mile (1.5K) easy 5 miles at 12:23 (8K at 7:42) 1 mile (1.5K) easy	15 miles at 13:08 (24K at 8:10)
14	1200 in 7:46 (200 RI); 1000 in 6:25 (200 RI); 800 in 5:06 (200 RI); 600 in 3:49 (200 RI); 400 in 2:32 (200 RI)	1 mile (1.5K) easy 5 miles at 11:32 (8K at 7:10) 1 mile (1.5K) easy	17 miles at 13:08 (27K at 8:10)
13	5 × 1000 in 6:25 (400 RI)	1 mile (1.5K) easy 4 miles at 11:17 (6.5K at 7:01) 1 mile (1.5K) easy	20 miles at 13:23 (32K at 8:19)
12	3 × 1600 in 10:30 (400 RI)	2 miles (3K) easy 3 miles at 11:02 (5K at 6:51) 1 mile (1.5K) easy	18 miles at 13:08 (29K at 8:10)
11	2 × 1200 in 7:46 (2 min RI); 4 × 800 in 5:06 (2 min RI)	1 mile (1.5K) easy 5 miles at 11:17 (8K at 7:01) 1 mile (1.5K) easy	20 miles at 13:08 (32K at 8:10)
10	6 × 800 in 5:06 (90 sec RI)	1 mile (1.5K) easy 6 miles at 11:32 (10K at 7:10) 1 mile (1.5K) easy	13 miles at 12:38 (21K at 7:51)
9	2 × (6 × 400 in 2:32) (90 sec RI) (2 min 30 sec RI between sets)	2 miles (3K) easy 3 miles at 11:02 (5K at 6:51) 1 mile (1.5K) easy	18 miles at 12:53 (29K at 8:01)
8	2 × 1600 in 10:30 (60 sec RI) 2 × 800 in 5:06 (60 sec RI)	1 mile (1.5K) easy 4 miles at 11:17 (6.5K at 7:01) 1 mile (1.5K) easy	20 miles at 12:53 (32K at 8:01)
7	3 × (2 × 1200 in 7:46) (2 min RI) (4 min RI between sets)	10 min warmup 10 miles at 12:23 (16K at 7:42) 10 min cooldown	15 miles at 12:43 (24K at 7:54)
6	1000 in 6:25; 2000 in 13:12; 1000 in 6:25; 1000 in 6:25 (400 RI)	1 mile (1.5K) easy 5 miles at 12:23 (8K at 7:42) 1 mile (1.5K) easy	20 miles at 12:53 (32K at 8:01)

WEEK	KEY RUN #1	KEY RUN #2	KEY RUN #3
5	3 × 1600 in 10:30 (400 RI)	10 min warmup 10 miles at 12:23 *(16K at 7:42)* 10 min cooldown	15 miles at 12:38 *(24K at 7:51)*
4	10 × 400 in 2:32 (400 RI)	10 min warmup 8 miles at 12:23 *(13K at 7:42)* 10 min cooldown	20 miles at 12:38 *(32K at 7:51)*
3	8 × 800 in 5:06 (90 sec RI)	1 mile *(1.5K)* easy 5 miles at 11:17 *(8K at 7:01)* 1 mile *(1.5K)* easy	13 miles at 12:23 *(21K at 7:42)*
2	5 × 1000 in 6:25 (400 RI)	2 miles *(3K)* easy 3 miles at 11:02 *(5K at 6:51)* 1 mile *(1.5K)* easy	10 miles at 12:23 *(16K at 7:42)*
1	6 × 400 in 2:32 (400 RI)	10 min warmup 3 miles at 12:23 *(5K at 7:42)* 10 min cooldown	MARATHON 26.2 miles at 12:23 *(42.2K at 7:42)*

ACKNOWLEDGMENTS

For more than 25 years I have had the pleasure and benefit of collaborating with Scott Murr and Ray Moss. Our unending conversations have enriched my understanding of human performance. Fifteen years after the three of us began discussing running and how to develop training programs that would be efficient, accessible, and effective, we proposed to the Furman University administration that a Running Institute be established. After our proposal was approved, we began offering lectures to the community and collecting data on runners. The demand for our lectures, coaching and testing became much greater in the second year. Those annually increasing demands have continued through the 8 years that FIRST has existed. Scott and Ray have continued to work toward meeting those requests for services with the same enthusiasm they demonstrated in our inaugural year. That contagious energy developed a synergy that has enabled FIRST to be recognized around the globe. My professional life has been brightened by my curious and trusty coauthors.

For more than 60 years I have relied on my big brother, Don. I would not have considered a revision of this book without his willingness to partner again in its development. As in the first edition, his editing and preparation of tables were an immense contribution. Don is really the book's fourth author. He was involved in discussions of every concept and idea and carefully reviewed every word of the book multiple times.

Amby Burfoot has not only been invaluable to FIRST for his guidance and wisdom, he has been a personal inspiration. Amby is among the most knowledgeable people in the world about running. It's a treat to visit with him and learn about the many facets of running. As any serious runner knows, Amby is incredibly talented, but you would absolutely never know that from talking with him. He is an intellectual who communicates well with the common man. His contributions to the running world are surpassed by no one. We are truly grateful to be his friend. We are also grateful to our editor Shannon Welch at Rodale Books.

Much of what we have learned for this revision has come from our FIRST running retreats. Those retreats have been enhanced by several FIRST retreat faculty. Mickey McCauley, the director of the FIRST high school cross-country camp, has been with FIRST since its inception. He is a USA Track and Field certified coach and provides e-coaching to FIRST clients.

Dr. Blaise Williams, professor and chair of the physical therapy department at East Carolina University, brings to our retreats the knowledge of a biomechanist who is an expert at gait analysis and the experience of a physical therapist who is an expert with lower limb injuries. That extraordinary combination of knowledge and experience provides every retreat participant with a special analysis.

As a senior at Furman University, Jill Lucas did an independent study project under my supervision that led to the creation of the FIRST running retreat. During her independent study, I recognized her organizational skills and enthusiasm for running. Five years later Jill is still a significant contributor to the retreats while earning a master's degree and working toward a doctorate in exercise physiology.

We rely on our dependable and ever-pleasant administrative assistant, Lonita Stegall, for communications with FIRST clients and the preparation of materials for our presentations and clinics.

FIRST is indebted to Stanford Jennings and New Balance. Stanford has been a longtime supporter of our programs by providing New Balance products for our staff, races, and retreats. New Balance also gave a copy of *Run Less, Run Faster* to all the participants at The Running Event, a convention for owners and managers of running specialty stores.

We have been fortunate to interact with runners from all six inhabited continents. It's been a joy to learn about their challenges and successes. Those interactions have shaped our ideas and our programs. We continue to strive to develop programs and offer services to promote running as a healthy, safe, and fun activity.

Bill Pierce

APPENDIX A

How to Calculate Paces

Runners' lives are complicated by the intersection of metric and English race distances and a Babylonian-era base-60 time system. Use these methods to simplify calculating your average race pace.

Changing race time into pace in minutes and seconds per mile:

Take your race time and convert it to total seconds. How? Multiply the number of hours (if any) by 3,600. Multiply minutes by 60. Add these two figures and then add the race-time seconds to that total. Examples: A marathon run in 3:47:23 equals 10,800 (3 × 3,600) + 2,820 (47 × 60) + 23 = 13,643 seconds. A 5-mile race run in 33:15 = 1,980 (33 × 60) + 15 = 1,995 seconds.

Divide the total number of seconds by the distance for the race in miles. If the race is a metric distance, you must find the mile equivalent for the distance. (See the chart below.) Examples from above: Marathon pace = 13,643 seconds/26.22 miles = 520.3 seconds per mile. Five-mile pace = 1,995 seconds/5 miles = 399 seconds per mile.

Convert the seconds per mile pace to minutes and seconds per mile by dividing by 60 and noting the remainder seconds. For the marathon pace: 520.3 seconds per mile/60 = 8 minutes 40.3 seconds per mile. For the 5-mile pace: 399 seconds per mile / 60 = 6 minutes 39 seconds per mile.

Changing race time into pace in minutes and seconds per kilometer:

Take your race time and convert it to total seconds. How? Multiply the number of hours (if any) by 3,600. Multiply minutes by 60. Add these two figures and then add the race-time seconds to that total. Examples: A marathon run in 3:47:23 equals 10,800 (3 × 3,600) + 2,820 (47 × 60) + 23 = 13,643 seconds. An 8K race run in 33:15 = 1980 (33 × 60) + 15 = 1,995 seconds.

Divide the total number of seconds by the distance for the race in kilometers. If the race is an English distance, you must find the metric equivalent for the distance. (See the chart below.) Examples from above: Marathon pace = 13,643 seconds/42.2 kilometers = 323.3 seconds per kilometer. 8K pace = 1995 seconds/8 kilometers = 249.4 seconds per kilometer.

Convert the seconds per kilometer pace to minutes and seconds per kilometer by dividing by 60 and noting the remainder seconds. For the marathon pace: 323.3 seconds per kilometer/60 = 5 minutes 23.3 seconds per kilometer. For the 8K pace: 249.4 seconds per kilometer/60 = 4 minutes 9.4 seconds per kilometer.

Distance Equivalents for Common Race Distances

MILES	KILOMETERS	KILOMETERS	MILES
1	1.609	1	.6214
5	8.045	5	3.107
8	12.872	8	4.971
10	16.090	10	6.214
13.109	21.095	15	9.321
15	24.135	20	12.427
20	32.180	Half-Marathon (21.095)	13.095
26.219	42.190	Marathon (42.190)	26.219

CALCULATIONS FOR TREADMILL AND GARMIN USERS
Changing pace in miles per hour to pace in minutes and seconds per mile:

Divide your pace in miles per hour into 60 to get pace in minutes. Convert fractional part to seconds.

Example: You are running on a treadmill and the pace is given as 8.9 mph. Divide 60 by 8.9 to yield 6.742 minutes per mile. Multiply .742 by 60 to yield 44 seconds. Your pace is 6 minutes 44 seconds per mile.

Changing pace in minutes and seconds per mile to pace in miles per hour:

Change seconds to decimal part of a minute and add to minutes. Then divide 60 by total.

The key run workout is to be run at 8:45 pace. Your treadmill displays only miles per hour. Divide 45 seconds by 60 seconds to yield .75. Add to 8 to get 8.75. Divide 60 by 8.75 to yield 6.9 mph.

Changing pace in kilometers per hour to pace in minutes and seconds per kilometer:

Divide your pace in kilometers per hour into 60 to get pace in minutes. Convert fractional part to seconds.

Example: You are running on a treadmill and the pace is given as 14.5 kph. Divide 60 by 14.5 to yield 4.14 minutes per kilometer. Multiply .14 by 60 to yield 8 seconds. Your pace is 4 minutes 8 seconds per kilometer.

Changing pace in minutes and seconds per kilometer to pace in kilometers per hour:

Change seconds to decimal part of a minute and add to minutes. Then divide 60 by total.

The key run workout is to be run at 5:23 pace. Your treadmill displays only kilometers per hour. Divide 23 seconds by 60 seconds to yield .383. Add to 5 to get 5.383. Divide 60 by 5.383 to yield 11.1 kph.

APPENDIX B

ROAD AGE STANDARDS WMA 2010

Road Age Standards in H:MM:SS WMA 2010

	FEMALE				MALE			
AGE	5K	10K	H. MAR	MARATHON	5K	10K	H. MAR	MARATHON
OC* SEC	888	1820	3950	8125	774	1611	3553	7495
OC*	0:14:48	0:30:20	1:05:50	2:15:25	0:12:54	0:26:51	0:59:13	2:04:55
30	0:14:48	0:30:21	1:05:51	2:15:28	0:12:56	0:26:55	0:59:13	2:04:55
31	0:14:49	0:30:22	1:05:54	2:15:39	0:12:58	0:26:59	0:59:13	2:04:55
32	0:14:50	0:30:24	1:06:00	2:15:56	0:13:00	0:27:04	0:59:14	2:04:55
33	0:14:52	0:30:28	1:06:07	2:16:20	0:13:03	0:27:10	0:59:19	2:04:55
34	0:14:54	0:30:32	1:06:16	2:16:51	0:13:07	0:27:17	0:59:27	2:04:55
35	0:14:57	0:30:38	1:06:28	2:17:30	0:13:11	0:27:26	0:59:40	2:04:55
36	0:15:00	0:30:44	1:06:42	2:18:15	0:13:16	0:27:36	0:59:57	2:05:03
37	0:15:03	0:30:51	1:06:58	2:19:09	0:13:21	0:27:47	1:00:18	2:05:25
38	0:15:08	0:31:00	1:07:17	2:20:11	0:13:27	0:28:00	1:00:44	2:06:03
39	0:15:12	0:31:10	1:07:38	2:21:20	0:13:33	0:28:12	1:01:12	2:06:57
40	0:15:18	0:31:21	1:08:01	2:22:39	0:13:39	0:28:25	1:01:41	2:08:00
41	0:15:23	0:31:32	1:08:27	2:24:07	0:13:45	0:28:37	1:02:11	2:09:04
42	0:15:30	0:31:46	1:08:56	2:25:44	0:13:51	0:28:50	1:02:41	2:10:08
43	0:15:37	0:32:00	1:09:27	2:27:28	0:13:58	0:29:04	1:03:11	2:11:14
44	0:15:44	0:32:16	1:10:01	2:29:14	0:14:04	0:29:17	1:03:42	2:12:20
45	0:15:53	0:32:33	1:10:39	2:31:03	0:14:11	0:29:31	1:04:13	2:13:29
46	0:16:02	0:32:51	1:11:19	2:32:55	0:14:17	0:29:44	1:04:45	2:14:38
47	0:16:12	0:33:11	1:12:02	2:34:49	0:14:24	0:29:58	1:05:17	2:15:49
48	0:16:22	0:33:33	1:12:49	2:36:46	0:14:31	0:30:13	1:05:50	2:17:00
49	0:16:34	0:33:56	1:13:40	2:38:46	0:14:38	0:30:27	1:06:23	2:18:13
50	0:16:46	0:34:22	1:14:34	2:40:50	0:14:45	0:30:42	1:06:57	2:19:28
51	0:16:58	0:34:47	1:15:30	2:42:56	0:14:52	0:30:57	1:07:32	2:20:43
52	0:17:11	0:35:14	1:16:28	2:45:06	0:14:59	0:31:12	1:08:07	2:22:00
53	0:17:25	0:35:41	1:17:27	2:47:20	0:15:07	0:31:27	1:08:43	2:23:18

	FEMALE				MALE			
AGE	**5K**	**10K**	**H. MAR**	**MARATHON**	**5K**	**10K**	**H. MAR**	**MARATHON**
OC* SEC	888	1820	3950	8125	774	1611	3553	7495
OC*	0:14:48	0:30:20	1:05:50	2:15:25	0:12:54	0:26:51	0:59:13	2:04:55
54	0:17:38	0:36:09	1:18:27	2:49:37	0:15:14	0:31:43	1:09:19	2:24:38
55	0:17:52	0:36:37	1:19:29	2:51:57	0:15:22	0:31:59	1:09:56	2:26:00
56	0:18:06	0:37:07	1:20:32	2:54:22	0:15:30	0:32:15	1:10:34	2:27:23
57	0:18:21	0:37:37	1:21:38	2:56:51	0:15:38	0:32:32	1:11:12	2:28:47
58	0:18:36	0:38:08	1:22:45	2:59:24	0:15:46	0:32:48	1:11:51	2:30:13
59	0:18:52	0:38:39	1:23:54	3:02:02	0:15:54	0:33:06	1:12:32	2:31:40
60	0:19:08	0:39:12	1:25:05	3:04:45	0:16:02	0:33:23	1:13:12	2:33:11
61	0:19:24	0:39:46	1:26:18	3:07:32	0:16:11	0:33:41	1:13:53	2:34:42
62	0:19:41	0:40:20	1:27:33	3:10:24	0:16:19	0:33:59	1:14:35	2:36:15
63	0:19:58	0:40:56	1:28:50	3:13:22	0:16:28	0:34:17	1:15:19	2:37:49
64	0:20:16	0:41:32	1:30:09	3:16:26	0:16:37	0:34:36	1:16:02	2:39:26
65	0:20:35	0:42:10	1:31:31	3:19:35	0:16:46	0:34:55	1:16:47	2:41:06
66	0:20:54	0:42:49	1:32:56	3:22:50	0:16:56	0:35:14	1:17:32	2:42:47
67	0:21:13	0:43:29	1:34:23	3:26:12	0:17:05	0:35:34	1:18:19	2:44:30
68	0:21:33	0:44:11	1:35:53	3:29:41	0:17:15	0:35:54	1:19:06	2:46:15
69	0:21:54	0:44:54	1:37:26	3:33:17	0:17:26	0:36:16	1:19:55	2:48:02
70	0:22:16	0:45:38	1:39:02	3:37:01	0:17:38	0:36:41	1:20:45	2:49:53
71	0:22:38	0:46:23	1:40:41	3:40:52	0:17:51	0:37:08	1:21:39	2:51:47
72	0:23:01	0:47:10	1:42:23	3:44:52	0:18:05	0:37:38	1:22:38	2:53:51
73	0:23:25	0:47:59	1:44:09	3:49:01	0:18:21	0:38:11	1:23:45	2:56:10
74	0:23:49	0:48:50	1:45:59	3:53:21	0:18:38	0:38:47	1:24:58	2:58:42
75	0:24:15	0:49:42	1:47:52	3:58:09	0:18:57	0:39:26	1:26:19	3:01:31
76	0:24:41	0:50:36	1:49:50	4:03:31	0:19:17	0:40:09	1:27:48	3:04:37
77	0:25:09	0:51:33	1:51:52	4:09:26	0:19:40	0:40:56	1:29:25	3:08:01
78	0:25:37	0:52:31	1:53:59	4:16:02	0:20:05	0:41:47	1:31:13	3:11:44
79	0:26:07	0:53:32	1:56:10	4:23:24	0:20:32	0:42:43	1:33:10	3:15:49
80	0:26:39	0:54:38	1:58:35	4:31:39	0:21:01	0:43:45	1:35:20	3:20:19
81	0:27:17	0:55:55	2:01:21	4:40:53	0:21:33	0:44:52	1:37:41	3:25:17
82	0:28:00	0:57:23	2:04:33	4:51:13	0:22:09	0:46:06	1:40:17	3:30:43
83	0:28:49	0:59:04	2:08:12	5:02:53	0:22:47	0:47:26	1:43:10	3:36:43
84	0:29:46	1:01:00	2:12:24	5:16:06	0:23:30	0:48:55	1:46:20	3:43:21
85	0:30:51	1:03:14	2:17:14	5:31:10	0:24:18	0:50:34	1:49:51	3:50:41

* All Masters standards/factors are as approved by the WMA Vice President

Non Stadia, WMA President, and USATF MLDR Committee

OC* Open-Class Standards represent the fastest time possible, at present, for a given distance.

APPENDIX C

ROAD AGE FACTORS
WMA 2010

Road Age Factors WMA 2010*

	FEMALE				MALE			
AGE	5K	10K	H. MAR	MARATHON	5K	10K	H. MAR	MARATHON
OC* SEC	888	1820	3950	8125	774	1611	3553	7495
OC*	0:14:48	0:30:20	1:05:50	2:15:25	0:12:54	0:26:51	0:59:13	2:04:55
30	0.9997	0.9997	0.9997	0.9996	0.9975	0.9975	1.0000	1.0000
31	0.9989	0.9989	0.9989	0.9983	0.9952	0.9952	1.0000	1.0000
32	0.9976	0.9976	0.9976	0.9962	0.9922	0.9922	0.9998	1.0000
33	0.9957	0.9957	0.9957	0.9933	0.9885	0.9885	0.9984	1.0000
34	0.9934	0.9934	0.9934	0.9895	0.9840	0.9840	0.9960	1.0000
35	0.9904	0.9904	0.9904	0.9849	0.9788	0.9788	0.9925	1.0000
36	0.9870	0.9870	0.9870	0.9795	0.9729	0.9729	0.9878	0.9990
37	0.9830	0.9830	0.9830	0.9732	0.9662	0.9662	0.9820	0.9960
38	0.9785	0.9785	0.9785	0.9660	0.9592	0.9592	0.9750	0.9910
39	0.9734	0.9734	0.9734	0.9581	0.9521	0.9521	0.9675	0.9840
40	0.9678	0.9678	0.9678	0.9493	0.9451	0.9451	0.9599	0.9759
41	0.9617	0.9617	0.9617	0.9396	0.9380	0.9380	0.9524	0.9679
42	0.9551	0.9551	0.9551	0.9292	0.9310	0.9310	0.9448	0.9599
43	0.9479	0.9479	0.9479	0.9183	0.9240	0.9240	0.9373	0.9519
44	0.9402	0.9402	0.9402	0.9074	0.9169	0.9169	0.9297	0.9439
45	0.9319	0.9319	0.9319	0.8965	0.9099	0.9099	0.9222	0.9358
46	0.9232	0.9232	0.9232	0.8856	0.9028	0.9028	0.9146	0.9278
47	0.9139	0.9139	0.9139	0.8747	0.8958	0.8958	0.9071	0.9198
48	0.9040	0.9040	0.9040	0.8638	0.8888	0.8888	0.8995	0.9118
49	0.8937	0.8937	0.8937	0.8529	0.8817	0.8817	0.8920	0.9038
50	0.8828	0.8828	0.8828	0.8420	0.8747	0.8747	0.8844	0.8957
51	0.8719	0.8719	0.8719	0.8311	0.8676	0.8676	0.8769	0.8877
52	0.8610	0.8610	0.8610	0.8202	0.8606	0.8606	0.8693	0.8797
53	0.8501	0.8501	0.8501	0.8093	0.8536	0.8536	0.8618	0.8717

	FEMALE				MALE			
AGE	5K	10K	H. MAR	MARATHON	5K	10K	H. MAR	MARATHON
OC* SEC	888	1820	3950	8125	774	1611	3553	7495
OC*	0:14:48	0:30:20	1:05:50	2:15:25	0:12:54	0:26:51	0:59:13	2:04:55
54	0.8392	0.8392	0.8392	0.7984	0.8465	0.8465	0.8542	0.8637
55	0.8283	0.8283	0.8283	0.7875	0.8395	0.8395	0.8467	0.8556
56	0.8174	0.8174	0.8174	0.7766	0.8324	0.8324	0.8392	0.8476
57	0.8065	0.8065	0.8065	0.7657	0.8254	0.8254	0.8316	0.8396
58	0.7956	0.7956	0.7956	0.7548	0.8184	0.8184	0.8241	0.8316
59	0.7847	0.7847	0.7847	0.7439	0.8113	0.8113	0.8165	0.8236
60	0.7738	0.7738	0.7738	0.7330	0.8043	0.8043	0.8090	0.8155
61	0.7629	0.7629	0.7629	0.7221	0.7972	0.7972	0.8014	0.8075
62	0.7520	0.7520	0.7520	0.7112	0.7902	0.7902	0.7939	0.7995
63	0.7411	0.7411	0.7411	0.7003	0.7832	0.7832	0.7863	0.7915
64	0.7302	0.7302	0.7302	0.6894	0.7761	0.7761	0.7788	0.7835
65	0.7193	0.7193	0.7193	0.6785	0.7691	0.7691	0.7712	0.7754
66	0.7084	0.7084	0.7084	0.6676	0.7620	0.7620	0.7637	0.7674
67	0.6975	0.6975	0.6975	0.6567	0.7550	0.7550	0.7561	0.7594
68	0.6866	0.6866	0.6866	0.6458	0.7479	0.7479	0.7486	0.7514
69	0.6757	0.6757	0.6757	0.6349	0.7402	0.7402	0.7410	0.7434
70	0.6648	0.6648	0.6648	0.6240	0.7319	0.7319	0.7334	0.7353
71	0.6539	0.6539	0.6539	0.6131	0.7230	0.7230	0.7253	0.7272
72	0.6430	0.6430	0.6430	0.6022	0.7134	0.7134	0.7166	0.7185
73	0.6321	0.6321	0.6321	0.5913	0.7031	0.7031	0.7071	0.7091
74	0.6212	0.6212	0.6212	0.5803	0.6923	0.6923	0.6969	0.6990
75	0.6103	0.6103	0.6103	0.5686	0.6808	0.6808	0.6860	0.6882
76	0.5994	0.5994	0.5994	0.5561	0.6687	0.6687	0.6744	0.6766
77	0.5885	0.5885	0.5885	0.5429	0.6559	0.6559	0.6622	0.6644
78	0.5776	0.5776	0.5776	0.5289	0.6425	0.6425	0.6492	0.6515
79	0.5667	0.5667	0.5667	0.5141	0.6285	0.6285	0.6356	0.6379
80	0.5552	0.5552	0.5552	0.4985	0.6138	0.6138	0.6212	0.6236
81	0.5425	0.5425	0.5425	0.4821	0.5985	0.5985	0.6062	0.6085
82	0.5286	0.5286	0.5286	0.4650	0.5825	0.5825	0.5905	0.5928
83	0.5135	0.5135	0.5135	0.4471	0.5660	0.5660	0.5740	0.5764
84	0.4972	0.4972	0.4972	0.4284	0.5488	0.5488	0.5569	0.5593
85	0.4797	0.4797	0.4797	0.4089	0.5309	0.5309	0.5391	0.5415

* All Masters standards/factors are as approved by the WMA Vice President

Non Stadia, WMA President, and USATF MLDR Committee

OC* Open-Class Standards represent the fastest time possible, at present, for a given distance.

APPENDIX D

PACE TABLES

Race Times for a Given Pace per Mile

MM:SS/MI	5K	10K	HALF-MARATHON	MARATHON
0:05:00	0:15:32	0:31:05	1:05:33	2:11:06
0:05:01	0:15:35	0:31:11	1:05:46	2:11:32
0:05:02	0:15:38	0:31:17	1:05:59	2:11:58
0:05:03	0:15:42	0:31:23	1:06:12	2:12:24
0:05:04	0:15:45	0:31:29	1:06:25	2:12:51
0:05:05	0:15:48	0:31:36	1:06:38	2:13:17
0:05:06	0:15:51	0:31:42	1:06:51	2:13:43
0:05:07	0:15:54	0:31:48	1:07:05	2:14:09
0:05:08	0:15:57	0:31:54	1:07:18	2:14:35
0:05:09	0:16:00	0:32:00	1:07:31	2:15:02
0:05:10	0:16:03	0:32:07	1:07:44	2:15:28
0:05:11	0:16:06	0:32:13	1:07:57	2:15:54
0:05:12	0:16:10	0:32:19	1:08:10	2:16:20
0:05:13	0:16:13	0:32:25	1:08:23	2:16:46
0:05:14	0:16:16	0:32:32	1:08:36	2:17:13
0:05:15	0:16:19	0:32:38	1:08:49	2:17:39
0:05:16	0:16:22	0:32:44	1:09:03	2:18:05
0:05:17	0:16:25	0:32:50	1:09:16	2:18:31
0:05:18	0:16:28	0:32:56	1:09:29	2:18:58
0:05:19	0:16:31	0:33:03	1:09:42	2:19:24
0:05:20	0:16:34	0:33:09	1:09:55	2:19:50
0:05:21	0:16:38	0:33:15	1:10:08	2:20:16
0:05:22	0:16:41	0:33:21	1:10:21	2:20:42
0:05:23	0:16:44	0:33:27	1:10:34	2:21:09
0:05:24	0:16:47	0:33:34	1:10:47	2:21:35
0:05:25	0:16:50	0:33:40	1:11:01	2:22:01
0:05:26	0:16:53	0:33:46	1:11:14	2:22:27
0:05:27	0:16:56	0:33:52	1:11:27	2:22:54
0:05:28	0:16:59	0:33:59	1:11:40	2:23:20
0:05:29	0:17:02	0:34:05	1:11:53	2:23:46

MM:SS/MI	5K	10K	HALF-MARATHON	MARATHON
0:05:30	0:17:05	0:34:11	1:12:06	2:24:12
0:05:31	0:17:09	0:34:17	1:12:19	2:24:38
0:05:32	0:17:12	0:34:23	1:12:32	2:25:05
0:05:33	0:17:15	0:34:30	1:12:45	2:25:31
0:05:34	0:17:18	0:34:36	1:12:59	2:25:57
0:05:35	0:17:21	0:34:42	1:13:12	2:26:23
0:05:36	0:17:24	0:34:48	1:13:25	2:26:50
0:05:37	0:17:27	0:34:54	1:13:38	2:27:16
0:05:38	0:17:30	0:35:01	1:13:51	2:27:42
0:05:39	0:17:33	0:35:07	1:14:04	2:28:08
0:05:40	0:17:37	0:35:13	1:14:17	2:28:34
0:05:41	0:17:40	0:35:19	1:14:30	2:29:01
0:05:42	0:17:43	0:35:26	1:14:43	2:29:27
0:05:43	0:17:46	0:35:32	1:14:57	2:29:53
0:05:44	0:17:49	0:35:38	1:15:10	2:30:19
0:05:45	0:17:52	0:35:44	1:15:23	2:30:45
0:05:46	0:17:55	0:35:50	1:15:36	2:31:12
0:05:47	0:17:58	0:35:57	1:15:49	2:31:38
0:05:48	0:18:01	0:36:03	1:16:02	2:32:04
0:05:49	0:18:05	0:36:09	1:16:15	2:32:30
0:05:50	0:18:08	0:36:15	1:16:28	2:32:57
0:05:51	0:18:11	0:36:21	1:16:41	2:33:23
0:05:52	0:18:14	0:36:28	1:16:54	2:33:49
0:05:53	0:18:17	0:36:34	1:17:08	2:34:15
0:05:54	0:18:20	0:36:40	1:17:21	2:34:41
0:05:55	0:18:23	0:36:46	1:17:34	2:35:08
0:05:56	0:18:26	0:36:53	1:17:47	2:35:34
0:05:57	0:18:29	0:36:59	1:18:00	2:36:00
0:05:58	0:18:32	0:37:05	1:18:13	2:36:26
0:05:59	0:18:36	0:37:11	1:18:26	2:36:53
0:06:00	0:18:39	0:37:17	1:18:39	2:37:19
0:06:01	0:18:42	0:37:24	1:18:52	2:37:45
0:06:02	0:18:45	0:37:30	1:19:06	2:38:11
0:06:03	0:18:48	0:37:36	1:19:19	2:38:37
0:06:04	0:18:51	0:37:42	1:19:32	2:39:04
0:06:05	0:18:54	0:37:48	1:19:45	2:39:30
0:06:06	0:18:57	0:37:55	1:19:58	2:39:56
0:06:07	0:19:00	0:38:01	1:20:11	2:40:22
0:06:08	0:19:04	0:38:07	1:20:24	2:40:48
0:06:09	0:19:07	0:38:13	1:20:37	2:41:15

MM:SS/MI	5K	10K	HALF-MARATHON	MARATHON
0:06:10	0:19:10	0:38:20	1:20:50	2:41:41
0:06:11	0:19:13	0:38:26	1:21:04	2:42:07
0:06:12	0:19:16	0:38:32	1:21:17	2:42:33
0:06:13	0:19:19	0:38:38	1:21:30	2:43:00
0:06:14	0:19:22	0:38:44	1:21:43	2:43:26
0:06:15	0:19:25	0:38:51	1:21:56	2:43:52
0:06:16	0:19:28	0:38:57	1:22:09	2:44:18
0:06:17	0:19:32	0:39:03	1:22:22	2:44:44
0:06:18	0:19:35	0:39:09	1:22:35	2:45:11
0:06:19	0:19:38	0:39:16	1:22:48	2:45:37
0:06:20	0:19:41	0:39:22	1:23:02	2:46:03
0:06:21	0:19:44	0:39:28	1:23:15	2:46:29
0:06:22	0:19:47	0:39:34	1:23:28	2:46:56
0:06:23	0:19:50	0:39:40	1:23:41	2:47:22
0:06:24	0:19:53	0:39:47	1:23:54	2:47:48
0:06:25	0:19:56	0:39:53	1:24:07	2:48:14
0:06:26	0:20:00	0:39:59	1:24:20	2:48:40
0:06:27	0:20:03	0:40:05	1:24:33	2:49:07
0:06:28	0:20:06	0:40:11	1:24:46	2:49:33
0:06:29	0:20:09	0:40:18	1:25:00	2:49:59
0:06:30	0:20:12	0:40:24	1:25:13	2:50:25
0:06:31	0:20:15	0:40:30	1:25:26	2:50:52
0:06:32	0:20:18	0:40:36	1:25:39	2:51:18
0:06:33	0:20:21	0:40:43	1:25:52	2:51:44
0:06:34	0:20:24	0:40:49	1:26:05	2:52:10
0:06:35	0:20:27	0:40:55	1:26:18	2:52:46
0:06:36	0:20:31	0:41:01	1:26:31	2:53:03
0:06:37	0:20:34	0:41:07	1:26:44	2:53:29
0:06:38	0:20:37	0:41:14	1:26:58	2:53:55
0:06:39	0:20:40	0:41:20	1:27:11	2:54:21
0:06:40	0:20:43	0:41:26	1:27:24	2:54:47
0:06:41	0:20:46	0:41:32	1:27:37	2:55:14
0:06:42	0:20:49	0:41:38	1:27:50	2:55:40
0:06:43	0:20:52	0:41:45	1:28:03	2:56:06
0:06:44	0:20:55	0:41:51	1:28:16	2:56:32
0:06:45	0:20:59	0:41:57	1:28:29	2:56:59
0:06:46	0:21:02	0:42:03	1:28:42	2:57:25
0:06:47	0:21:05	0:42:10	1:28:56	2:57:51
0:06:48	0:21:08	0:42:16	1:29:09	2:58:17
0:06:49	0:21:11	0:42:22	1:29:22	2:58:43

MM:SS/MI	5K	10K	HALF-MARATHON	MARATHON
0:06:50	0:21:14	0:42:28	1:29:35	2:59:10
0:06:51	0:21:17	0:42:34	1:29:48	2:59:36
0:06:52	0:21:20	0:42:41	1:30:01	3:00:02
0:06:53	0:21:23	0:42:47	1:30:14	3:00:28
0:06:54	0:21:27	0:42:53	1:30:27	3:00:55
0:06:55	0:21:30	0:42:59	1:30:40	3:01:21
0:06:56	0:21:33	0:43:05	1:30:53	3:01:47
0:06:57	0:21:36	0:43:12	1:31:07	3:02:13
0:06:58	0:21:39	0:43:18	1:31:20	3:02:39
0:06:59	0:21:42	0:43:24	1:31:33	3:03:06
0:07:00	0:21:45	0:43:30	1:31:46	3:03:32
0:07:01	0:21:48	0:43:37	1:31:59	3:03:58
0:07:02	0:21:51	0:43:43	1:32:12	3:04:24
0:07:03	0:21:54	0:43:49	1:32:25	3:04:51
0:07:04	0:21:58	0:43:55	1:32:38	3:05:17
0:07:05	0:22:01	0:44:01	1:32:51	3:05:43
0:07:06	0:22:04	0:44:08	1:33:05	3:06:09
0:07:07	0:22:07	0:44:14	1:33:18	3:06:35
0:07:08	0:22:10	0:44:20	1:33:31	3:07:02
0:07:09	0:22:13	0:44:26	1:33:44	3:07:28
0:07:10	0:22:16	0:44:32	1:33:57	3:07:54
0:07:11	0:22:19	0:44:39	1:34:10	3:08:20
0:07:12	0:22:22	0:44:45	1:34:23	3:08:46
0:07:13	0:22:26	0:44:51	1:34:36	3:09:13
0:07:14	0:22:29	0:44:57	1:34:49	3:09:39
0:07:15	0:22:32	0:45:04	1:35:03	3:10:05
0:07:16	0:22:35	0:45:10	1:35:16	3:10:31
0:07:17	0:22:38	0:45:16	1:35:29	3:10:58
0:07:18	0:22:41	0:45:22	1:35:42	3:11:24
0:07:19	0:22:44	0:45:28	1:35:55	3:11:50
0:07:20	0:22:47	0:45:35	1:36:08	3:12:16
0:07:21	0:22:50	0:45:41	1:36:21	3:12:42
0:07:22	0:22:54	0:45:47	1:36:34	3:13:09
0:07:23	0:22:57	0:45:53	1:36:47	3:13:35
0:07:24	0:23:00	0:45:59	1:37:01	3:14:01
0:07:25	0:23:03	0:46:06	1:37:14	3:14:27
0:07:26	0:23:06	0:46:12	1:37:27	3:14:54
0:07:27	0:23:09	0:46:18	1:37:40	3:15:20
0:07:28	0:23:12	0:46:24	1:37:53	3:15:46
0:07:29	0:23:15	0:46:31	1:38:06	3:16:12

MM:SS/MI	5K	10K	HALF-MARATHON	MARATHON
0:07:30	0:23:18	0:46:37	1:38:19	3:16:38
0:07:31	0:23:21	0:46:43	1:38:32	3:17:05
0:07:32	0:23:25	0:46:49	1:38:45	3:17:31
0:07:33	0:23:28	0:46:55	1:38:59	3:17:57
0:07:34	0:23:31	0:47:02	1:39:12	3:18:23
0:07:35	0:23:34	0:47:08	1:39:25	3:18:50
0:07:36	0:23:37	0:47:14	1:39:38	3:19:16
0:07:37	0:23:40	0:47:20	1:39:51	3:19:42
0:07:38	0:23:43	0:47:26	1:40:04	3:20:08
0:07:39	0:23:46	0:47:33	1:40:17	3:20:34
0:07:40	0:23:49	0:47:39	1:40:30	3:21:01
0:07:41	0:23:53	0:47:45	1:40:43	3:21:27
0:07:42	0:23:56	0:47:51	1:40:57	3:21:53
0:07:43	0:23:59	0:47:58	1:41:10	3:22:19
0:07:44	0:24:02	0:48:04	1:41:23	3:22:45
0:07:45	0:24:05	0:48:10	1:41:36	3:23:12
0:07:46	0:24:08	0:48:16	1:41:49	3:23:38
0:07:47	0:24:11	0:48:22	1:42:02	3:24:04
0:07:48	0:24:14	0:48:29	1:42:15	3:24:30
0:07:49	0:24:17	0:48:35	1:42:28	3:24:57
0:07:50	0:24:21	0:48:41	1:42:41	3:25:23
0:07:51	0:24:24	0:48:47	1:42:55	3:25:49
0:07:52	0:24:27	0:48:53	1:43:08	3:26:15
0:07:53	0:24:30	0:49:00	1:43:21	3:26:41
0:07:54	0:24:33	0:49:06	1:43:34	3:27:08
0:07:55	0:24:36	0:49:12	1:43:47	3:27:34
0:07:56	0:24:39	0:49:18	1:44:00	3:28:00
0:07:57	0:24:42	0:49:25	1:44:13	3:28:26
0:07:58	0:24:45	0:49:31	1:44:26	3:28:53
0:07:59	0:24:49	0:49:37	1:44:39	3:29:19
0:08:00	0:24:52	0:49:43	1:44:52	3:29:45
0:08:01	0:24:55	0:49:49	1:45:06	3:30:11
0:08:02	0:24:58	0:49:56	1:45:19	3:30:37
0:08:03	0:25:01	0:50:02	1:45:32	3:31:04
0:08:04	0:25:04	0:50:08	1:45:45	3:31:30
0:08:05	0:25:07	0:50:14	1:45:58	3:31:56
0:08:06	0:25:10	0:50:21	1:46:11	3:32:22
0:08:07	0:25:13	0:50:27	1:46:24	3:32:49
0:08:08	0:25:16	0:50:33	1:46:37	3:33:15
0:08:09	0:25:20	0:50:39	1:46:50	3:33:41

MM:SS/MI	5K	10K	HALF-MARATHON	MARATHON
0:08:10	0:25:23	0:50:45	1:47:04	3:34:07
0:08:11	0:25:26	0:50:52	1:47:17	3:34:33
0:08:12	0:25:29	0:50:58	1:47:30	3:35:00
0:08:13	0:25:32	0:51:04	1:47:43	3:35:26
0:08:14	0:25:35	0:51:10	1:47:56	3:35:52
0:08:15	0:25:38	0:51:16	1:48:09	3:36:18
0:08:16	0:25:41	0:51:23	1:48:22	3:36:44
0:08:17	0:25:44	0:51:29	1:48:35	3:37:11
0:08:18	0:25:48	0:51:35	1:48:48	3:37:37
0:08:19	0:25:51	0:51:41	1:49:02	3:38:03
0:08:20	0:25:54	0:51:48	1:49:15	3:38:29
0:08:21	0:25:57	0:51:54	1:49:28	3:38:56
0:08:22	0:26:00	0:52:00	1:49:41	3:39:22
0:08:23	0:26:03	0:52:06	1:49:54	3:39:48
0:08:24	0:26:06	0:52:12	1:50:07	3:40:14
0:08:25	0:26:09	0:52:19	1:50:20	3:40:40
0:08:26	0:26:12	0:52:25	1:50:33	3:41:07
0:08:27	0:26:16	0:52:31	1:50:46	3:41:33
0:08:28	0:26:19	0:52:37	1:51:00	3:41:59
0:08:29	0:26:22	0:52:43	1:51:13	3:42:25
0:08:30	0:26:25	0:52:50	1:51:26	3:42:52
0:08:31	0:26:28	0:52:56	1:51:39	3:43:18
0:08:32	0:26:31	0:53:02	1:51:52	3:43:44
0:08:33	0:26:34	0:53:08	1:52:05	3:44:10
0:08:34	0:26:37	0:53:15	1:52:18	3:44:36
0:08:35	0:26:40	0:53:21	1:52:31	3:45:03
0:08:36	0:26:43	0:53:27	1:52:44	3:45:29
0:08:37	0:26:47	0:53:33	1:52:58	3:45:55
0:08:38	0:26:50	0:53:39	1:53:11	3:46:21
0:08:39	0:26:53	0:53:46	1:53:24	3:46:48
0:08:40	0:26:56	0:53:52	1:53:37	3:47:14
0:08:41	0:26:59	0:53:58	1:53:50	3:47:40
0:08:42	0:27:02	0:54:04	1:54:03	3:48:06
0:08:43	0:27:05	0:54:10	1:54:16	3:48:32
0:08:44	0:27:08	0:54:17	1:54:29	3:48:59
0:08:45	0:27:11	0:54:23	1:54:42	3:49:25
0:08:46	0:27:15	0:54:29	1:54:56	3:49:51
0:08:47	0:27:18	0:54:35	1:55:09	3:50:17
0:08:48	0:27:21	0:54:42	1:55:22	3:50:43
0:08:49	0:27:24	0:54:48	1:55:35	3:51:10

MM:SS/MI	5K	10K	HALF-MARATHON	MARATHON
0:08:50	0:27:27	0:54:54	1:55:48	3:51:36
0:08:51	0:27:30	0:55:00	1:56:01	3:52:02
0:08:52	0:27:33	0:55:06	1:56:14	3:52:28
0:08:53	0:27:36	0:55:13	1:56:27	3:52:55
0:08:54	0:27:39	0:55:19	1:56:40	3:53:21
0:08:55	0:27:43	0:55:25	1:56:54	3:53:47
0:08:56	0:27:46	0:55:31	1:57:07	3:54:13
0:08:57	0:27:49	0:55:37	1:57:20	3:54:39
0:08:58	0:27:52	0:55:44	1:57:33	3:55:06
0:08:59	0:27:55	0:55:50	1:57:46	3:55:32
0:09:00	0:27:58	0:55:56	1:57:59	3:55:58
0:09:01	0:28:01	0:56:02	1:58:12	3:56:24
0:09:02	0:28:04	0:56:09	1:58:25	3:56:51
0:09:03	0:28:07	0:56:15	1:58:38	3:57:17
0:09:04	0:28:10	0:56:21	1:58:51	3:57:43
0:09:05	0:28:14	0:56:27	1:59:05	3:58:09
0:09:06	0:28:17	0:56:33	1:59:18	3:58:35
0:09:07	0:28:20	0:56:40	1:59:31	3:59:02
0:09:08	0:28:23	0:56:46	1:59:44	3:59:28
0:09:09	0:28:26	0:56:52	1:59:57	3:59:54
0:09:10	0:28:29	0:56:58	2:00:10	4:00:20
0:09:11	0:28:32	0:57:04	2:00:23	4:00:47
0:09:12	0:28:35	0:57:11	2:00:36	4:01:13
0:09:13	0:28:38	0:57:17	2:00:49	4:01:39
0:09:14	0:28:42	0:57:23	2:01:03	4:02:05
0:09:15	0:28:45	0:57:29	2:01:16	4:02:31
0:09:16	0:28:48	0:57:36	2:01:29	4:02:58
0:09:17	0:28:51	0:57:42	2:01:42	4:03:24
0:09:18	0:28:54	0:57:48	2:01:55	4:03:50
0:09:19	0:28:57	0:57:54	2:02:08	4:04:16
0:09:20	0:29:00	0:58:00	2:02:21	4:04:42
0:09:21	0:29:03	0:58:07	2:02:34	4:05:09
0:09:22	0:29:06	0:58:13	2:02:47	4:05:35
0:09:23	0:29:10	0:58:19	2:03:01	4:06:01
0:09:24	0:29:13	0:58:25	2:03:14	4:06:27
0:09:25	0:29:16	0:58:31	2:03:27	4:06:54
0:09:26	0:29:19	0:58:38	2:03:40	4:07:20
0:09:27	0:29:22	0:58:44	2:03:53	4:07:46
0:09:28	0:29:25	0:58:50	2:04:06	4:08:12
0:09:29	0:29:28	0:58:56	2:04:19	4:08:38

MM:SS/MI	5K	10K	HALF-MARATHON	MARATHON
0:09:30	0:29:31	0:59:03	2:04:32	4:09:05
0:09:31	0:29:34	0:59:09	2:04:45	4:09:31
0:09:32	0:29:38	0:59:15	2:04:59	4:09:57
0:09:33	0:29:41	0:59:21	2:05:12	4:10:23
0:09:34	0:29:44	0:59:27	2:05:25	4:10:50
0:09:35	0:29:47	0:59:34	2:05:38	4:11:16
0:09:36	0:29:50	0:59:40	2:05:51	4:11:42
0:09:37	0:29:53	0:59:46	2:06:04	4:12:08
0:09:38	0:29:56	0:59:52	2:06:17	4:12:34
0:09:39	0:29:59	0:59:59	2:06:30	4:13:01
0:09:40	0:30:02	1:00:05	2:06:43	4:13:27
0:09:41	0:30:05	1:00:11	2:06:57	4:13:53
0:09:42	0:30:09	1:00:17	2:07:10	4:14:19
0:09:43	0:30:12	1:00:23	2:07:23	4:14:46
0:09:44	0:30:15	1:00:30	2:07:36	4:15:12
0:09:45	0:30:18	1:00:36	2:07:49	4:15:38
0:09:46	0:30:21	1:00:42	2:08:02	4:16:04
0:09:47	0:30:24	1:00:48	2:08:15	4:16:30
0:09:48	0:30:27	1:00:54	2:08:28	4:16:57
0:09:49	0:30:30	1:01:01	2:08:41	4:17:23
0:09:50	0:30:33	1:01:07	2:08:55	4:17:49
0:09:51	0:30:37	1:01:13	2:09:08	4:18:15
0:09:52	0:30:40	1:01:19	2:09:21	4:18:41
0:09:53	0:30:43	1:01:26	2:09:34	4:19:08
0:09:54	0:30:46	1:01:32	2:09:47	4:19:34
0:09:55	0:30:49	1:01:38	2:10:00	4:20:00
0:09:56	0:30:52	1:01:44	2:10:13	4:20:26
0:09:57	0:30:55	1:01:50	2:10:26	4:20:53
0:09:58	0:30:58	1:01:57	2:10:39	4:21:19
0:09:59	0:31:01	1:02:03	2:10:53	4:21:45
0:10:00	0:31:05	1:02:09	2:11:06	4:22:11
0:10:01	0:31:08	1:02:15	2:11:19	4:22:37
0:10:02	0:31:11	1:02:21	2:11:32	4:23:04
0:10:03	0:31:14	1:02:28	2:11:45	4:23:30
0:10:04	0:31:17	1:02:34	2:11:58	4:23:56
0:10:05	0:31:20	1:02:40	2:12:11	4:24:22
0:10:06	0:31:23	1:02:46	2:12:24	4:24:49
0:10:07	0:31:26	1:02:53	2:12:37	4:25:15
0:10:08	0:31:29	1:02:59	2:12:50	4:25:41
0:10:09	0:31:32	1:03:05	2:13:04	4:26:07

MM:SS/MI	5K	10K	HALF-MARATHON	MARATHON
0:10:10	0:31:36	1:03:11	2:13:17	4:26:33
0:10:11	0:31:39	1:03:17	2:13:30	4:27:00
0:10:12	0:31:42	1:03:24	2:13:43	4:27:26
0:10:13	0:31:45	1:03:30	2:13:56	4:27:52
0:10:14	0:31:48	1:03:36	2:14:09	4:28:18
0:10:15	0:31:51	1:03:42	2:14:22	4:28:45
0:10:16	0:31:54	1:03:48	2:14:35	4:29:11
0:10:17	0:31:57	1:03:55	2:14:48	4:29:37
0:10:18	0:32:00	1:04:01	2:15:02	4:30:03
0:10:19	0:32:04	1:04:07	2:15:15	4:30:29
0:10:20	0:32:07	1:04:13	2:15:28	4:30:56
0:10:21	0:32:10	1:04:20	2:15:41	4:31:22
0:10:22	0:32:13	1:04:26	2:15:54	4:31:48
0:10:23	0:32:16	1:04:32	2:16:07	4:32:14
0:10:24	0:32:19	1:04:38	2:16:20	4:32:40
0:10:25	0:32:22	1:04:44	2:16:33	4:33:07
0:10:26	0:32:25	1:04:51	2:16:46	4:33:33
0:10:27	0:32:28	1:04:57	2:17:00	4:33:59
0:10:28	0:32:32	1:05:03	2:17:13	4:34:25
0:10:29	0:32:35	1:05:09	2:17:26	4:34:52
0:10:30	0:32:38	1:05:15	2:17:39	4:35:18
0:10:31	0:32:41	1:05:22	2:17:52	4:35:44
0:10:32	0:32:44	1:05:28	2:18:05	4:36:10
0:10:33	0:32:47	1:05:34	2:18:18	4:36:36
0:10:34	0:32:50	1:05:40	2:18:31	4:37:03
0:10:35	0:32:53	1:05:47	2:18:44	4:37:29
0:10:36	0:32:56	1:05:53	2:18:58	4:37:55
0:10:37	0:32:59	1:05:59	2:19:11	4:38:21
0:10:38	0:33:03	1:06:05	2:19:24	4:38:48
0:10:39	0:33:06	1:06:11	2:19:37	4:39:14
0:10:40	0:33:09	1:06:18	2:19:50	4:39:40
0:10:41	0:33:12	1:06:24	2:20:03	4:40:06
0:10:42	0:33:15	1:06:30	2:20:16	4:40:32
0:10:43	0:33:18	1:06:36	2:20:29	4:40:59
0:10:44	0:33:21	1:06:42	2:20:42	4:41:25
0:10:45	0:33:24	1:06:49	2:20:56	4:41:51
0:10:46	0:33:27	1:06:55	2:21:09	4:42:17
0:10:47	0:33:31	1:07:01	2:21:22	4:42:44
0:10:48	0:33:34	1:07:07	2:21:35	4:43:10
0:10:49	0:33:37	1:07:14	2:21:48	4:43:36

MM:SS/MI	5K	10K	HALF-MARATHON	MARATHON
0:10:50	0:33:40	1:07:20	2:22:01	4:44:02
0:10:51	0:33:43	1:07:26	2:22:14	4:44:28
0:10:52	0:33:46	1:07:32	2:22:27	4:44:55
0:10:53	0:33:49	1:07:38	2:22:40	4:45:21
0:10:54	0:33:52	1:07:45	2:22:54	4:45:47
0:10:55	0:33:55	1:07:51	2:23:07	4:46:13
0:10:56	0:33:59	1:07:57	2:23:20	4:46:39
0:10:57	0:34:02	1:08:03	2:23:33	4:47:06
0:10:58	0:34:05	1:08:09	2:23:46	4:47:32
0:10:59	0:34:08	1:08:16	2:23:59	4:47:58
0:11:00	0:34:11	1:08:22	2:24:12	4:48:24
0:11:01	0:34:14	1:08:28	2:24:25	4:48:51
0:11:02	0:34:17	1:08:34	2:24:38	4:49:17
0:11:03	0:34:20	1:08:41	2:24:52	4:49:43
0:11:04	0:34:23	1:08:47	2:25:05	4:50:09
0:11:05	0:34:27	1:08:53	2:25:18	4:50:35
0:11:06	0:34:30	1:08:59	2:25:31	4:51:02
0:11:07	0:34:33	1:09:05	2:25:44	4:51:28
0:11:08	0:34:36	1:09:12	2:25:57	4:51:54
0:11:09	0:34:39	1:09:18	2:26:10	4:52:20
0:11:10	0:34:42	1:09:24	2:26:23	4:52:47
0:11:11	0:34:45	1:09:30	2:26:36	4:53:13
0:11:12	0:34:48	1:09:37	2:26:49	4:53:39
0:11:13	0:34:51	1:09:43	2:27:03	4:54:05
0:11:14	0:34:54	1:09:49	2:27:16	4:54:31
0:11:15	0:34:58	1:09:55	2:27:29	4:54:58
0:11:16	0:35:01	1:10:01	2:27:42	4:55:24
0:11:17	0:35:04	1:10:08	2:27:55	4:55:50
0:11:18	0:35:07	1:10:14	2:28:08	4:56:16
0:11:19	0:35:10	1:10:20	2:28:21	4:56:43
0:11:20	0:35:13	1:10:26	2:28:34	4:57:09
0:11:21	0:35:16	1:10:32	2:28:47	4:57:35
0:11:22	0:35:19	1:10:39	2:29:01	4:58:01
0:11:23	0:35:22	1:10:45	2:29:14	4:58:27
0:11:24	0:35:26	1:10:51	2:29:27	4:58:54
0:11:25	0:35:29	1:10:57	2:29:40	4:59:20
0:11:26	0:35:32	1:11:04	2:29:53	4:59:46
0:11:27	0:35:35	1:11:10	2:30:06	5:00:12
0:11:28	0:35:38	1:11:16	2:30:19	5:00:38
0:11:29	0:35:41	1:11:22	2:30:32	5:01:05

MM:SS/MI	5K	10K	HALF-MARATHON	MARATHON
0:11:30	0:35:44	1:11:28	2:30:45	5:01:31
0:11:31	0:35:47	1:11:35	2:30:59	5:01:57
0:11:32	0:35:50	1:11:41	2:31:12	5:02:23
0:11:33	0:35:54	1:11:47	2:31:25	5:02:50
0:11:34	0:35:57	1:11:53	2:31:38	5:03:16
0:11:35	0:36:00	1:11:59	2:31:51	5:03:42
0:11:36	0:36:03	1:12:06	2:32:04	5:04:08
0:11:37	0:36:06	1:12:12	2:32:17	5:04:34
0:11:38	0:36:09	1:12:18	2:32:30	5:05:01
0:11:39	0:36:12	1:12:24	2:32:43	5:05:27
0:11:40	0:36:15	1:12:31	2:32:57	5:05:53
0:11:41	0:36:18	1:12:37	2:33:10	5:06:19
0:11:42	0:36:21	1:12:43	2:33:23	5:06:46
0:11:43	0:36:25	1:12:49	2:33:36	5:07:12
0:11:44	0:36:28	1:12:55	2:33:49	5:07:38
0:11:45	0:36:31	1:13:02	2:34:02	5:08:04
0:11:46	0:36:34	1:13:08	2:34:15	5:08:30
0:11:47	0:36:37	1:13:14	2:34:28	5:08:57
0:11:48	0:36:40	1:13:20	2:34:41	5:09:23
0:11:49	0:36:43	1:13:26	2:34:55	5:09:49
0:11:50	0:36:46	1:13:33	2:35:08	5:10:15
0:11:51	0:36:49	1:13:39	2:35:21	5:10:42
0:11:52	0:36:53	1:13:45	2:35:34	5:11:08
0:11:53	0:36:56	1:13:51	2:35:47	5:11:34
0:11:54	0:36:59	1:13:58	2:36:00	5:12:00
0:11:55	0:37:02	1:14:04	2:36:13	5:12:26
0:11:56	0:37:05	1:14:10	2:36:26	5:12:53
0:11:57	0:37:08	1:14:16	2:36:39	5:13:19
0:11:58	0:37:11	1:14:22	2:36:53	5:13:45
0:11:59	0:37:14	1:14:29	2:37:06	5:14:11
0:12:00	0:37:17	1:14:35	2:37:19	5:14:37
0:12:01	0:37:21	1:14:41	2:37:32	5:15:04
0:12:02	0:37:24	1:14:47	2:37:45	5:15:30
0:12:03	0:37:27	1:14:53	2:37:58	5:15:56
0:12:04	0:37:30	1:15:00	2:38:11	5:16:22
0:12:05	0:37:33	1:15:06	2:38:24	5:16:49
0:12:06	0:37:36	1:15:12	2:38:37	5:17:15
0:12:07	0:37:39	1:15:18	2:38:51	5:17:41
0:12:08	0:37:42	1:15:25	2:39:04	5:18:07
0:12:09	0:37:45	1:15:31	2:39:17	5:18:33

MM:SS/MI	5K	10K	HALF-MARATHON	MARATHON
0:12:10	0:37:48	1:15:37	2:39:30	5:19:00
0:12:11	0:37:52	1:15:43	2:39:43	5:19:26
0:12:12	0:37:55	1:15:49	2:39:56	5:19:52
0:12:13	0:37:58	1:15:56	2:40:09	5:20:18
0:12:14	0:38:01	1:16:02	2:40:22	5:20:45
0:12:15	0:38:04	1:16:08	2:40:35	5:21:11
0:12:16	0:38:07	1:16:14	2:40:48	5:21:37
0:12:17	0:38:10	1:16:20	2:41:02	5:22:03
0:12:18	0:38:13	1:16:27	2:41:15	5:22:29
0:12:19	0:38:16	1:16:33	2:41:28	5:22:56
0:12:20	0:38:20	1:16:39	2:41:41	5:23:22
0:12:21	0:38:23	1:16:45	2:41:54	5:23:48
0:12:22	0:38:26	1:16:52	2:42:07	5:24:14
0:12:23	0:38:29	1:16:58	2:42:20	5:24:41
0:12:24	0:38:32	1:17:04	2:42:33	5:25:07
0:12:25	0:38:35	1:17:10	2:42:46	5:25:33
0:12:26	0:38:38	1:17:16	2:43:00	5:25:59
0:12:27	0:38:41	1:17:23	2:43:13	5:26:25
0:12:28	0:38:44	1:17:29	2:43:26	5:26:52
0:12:29	0:38:48	1:17:35	2:43:39	5:27:18
0:12:30	0:38:51	1:17:41	2:43:52	5:27:44
0:12:31	0:38:54	1:17:47	2:44:05	5:28:10
0:12:32	0:38:57	1:17:54	2:44:18	5:28:36
0:12:33	0:39:00	1:18:00	2:44:31	5:29:03
0:12:34	0:39:03	1:18:06	2:44:44	5:29:29
0:12:35	0:39:06	1:18:12	2:44:58	5:29:55
0:12:36	0:39:09	1:18:19	2:45:11	5:30:21
0:12:37	0:39:12	1:18:25	2:45:24	5:30:48
0:12:38	0:39:16	1:18:31	2:45:37	5:31:14
0:12:39	0:39:19	1:18:37	2:45:50	5:31:40
0:12:40	0:39:22	1:18:43	2:46:03	5:32:06
0:12:41	0:39:25	1:18:50	2:46:16	5:32:32
0:12:42	0:39:28	1:18:56	2:46:29	5:32:59
0:12:43	0:39:31	1:19:02	2:46:42	5:33:25
0:12:44	0:39:34	1:19:08	2:46:56	5:33:51
0:12:45	0:39:37	1:19:15	2:47:09	5:34:17
0:12:46	0:39:40	1:19:21	2:47:22	5:34:44
0:12:47	0:39:43	1:19:27	2:47:35	5:35:10
0:12:48	0:39:47	1:19:33	2:47:48	5:35:36
0:12:49	0:39:50	1:19:39	2:48:01	5:36:02

MM:SS/MI	5K	10K	HALF-MARATHON	MARATHON
0:12:50	0:39:53	1:19:46	2:48:14	5:36:28
0:12:51	0:39:56	1:19:52	2:48:27	5:36:55
0:12:52	0:39:59	1:19:58	2:48:40	5:37:21
0:12:53	0:40:02	1:20:04	2:48:54	5:37:47
0:12:54	0:40:05	1:20:10	2:49:07	5:38:13
0:12:55	0:40:08	1:20:17	2:49:20	5:38:40
0:12:56	0:40:11	1:20:23	2:49:33	5:39:06
0:12:57	0:40:15	1:20:29	2:49:46	5:39:32

Race Times for a Given Pace per Kilometer

MM:SS/KM	5K	10K	HALF-MARATHON	MARATHON
0:03:06	0:15:30	0:31:00	1:05:23	2:10:47
0:03:07	0:15:35	0:31:10	1:05:44	2:11:29
0:03:08	0:15:40	0:31:20	1:06:05	2:12:11
0:03:09	0:15:45	0:31:30	1:06:27	2:12:53
0:03:10	0:15:50	0:31:40	1:06:48	2:13:35
0:03:11	0:15:55	0:31:50	1:07:09	2:14:18
0:03:12	0:16:00	0:32:00	1:07:30	2:15:00
0:03:13	0:16:05	0:32:10	1:07:51	2:15:42
0:03:14	0:16:10	0:32:20	1:08:12	2:16:24
0:03:15	0:16:15	0:32:30	1:08:33	2:17:06
0:03:16	0:16:20	0:32:40	1:08:54	2:17:48
0:03:17	0:16:25	0:32:50	1:09:15	2:18:31
0:03:18	0:16:30	0:33:00	1:09:36	2:19:13
0:03:19	0:16:35	0:33:10	1:09:58	2:19:55
0:03:20	0:16:40	0:33:20	1:10:19	2:20:37
0:03:21	0:16:45	0:33:30	1:10:40	2:21:19
0:03:22	0:16:50	0:33:40	1:11:01	2:22:02
0:03:23	0:16:55	0:33:50	1:11:22	2:22:44
0:03:24	0:17:00	0:34:00	1:11:43	2:23:26
0:03:25	0:17:05	0:34:10	1:12:04	2:24:08
0:03:26	0:17:10	0:34:20	1:12:25	2:24:50
0:03:27	0:17:15	0:34:30	1:12:46	2:25:33
0:03:28	0:17:20	0:34:40	1:13:07	2:26:15
0:03:29	0:17:25	0:34:50	1:13:28	2:26:57
0:03:30	0:17:30	0:35:00	1:13:50	2:27:39
0:03:31	0:17:35	0:35:10	1:14:11	2:28:21
0:03:32	0:17:40	0:35:20	1:14:32	2:29:03
0:03:33	0:17:45	0:35:30	1:14:53	2:29:46
0:03:34	0:17:50	0:35:40	1:15:14	2:30:28
0:03:35	0:17:55	0:35:50	1:15:35	2:31:10
0:03:36	0:18:00	0:36:00	1:15:56	2:31:52
0:03:37	0:18:05	0:36:10	1:16:17	2:32:34
0:03:38	0:18:10	0:36:20	1:16:38	2:33:17
0:03:39	0:18:15	0:36:30	1:16:59	2:33:59
0:03:40	0:18:20	0:36:40	1:17:20	2:34:41
0:03:41	0:18:25	0:36:50	1:17:42	2:35:23
0:03:42	0:18:30	0:37:00	1:18:03	2:36:05
0:03:43	0:18:35	0:37:10	1:18:24	2:36:47

MM:SS/KM	5K	10K	HALF-MARATHON	MARATHON
0:03:44	0:18:40	0:37:20	1:18:45	2:37:30
0:03:45	0:18:45	0:37:30	1:19:06	2:38:12
0:03:46	0:18:50	0:37:40	1:19:27	2:38:54
0:03:47	0:18:55	0:37:50	1:19:48	2:39:36
0:03:48	0:19:00	0:38:00	1:20:09	2:40:18
0:03:49	0:19:05	0:38:10	1:20:30	2:41:01
0:03:50	0:19:10	0:38:20	1:20:51	2:41:43
0:03:51	0:19:15	0:38:30	1:21:12	2:42:25
0:03:52	0:19:20	0:38:40	1:21:34	2:43:07
0:03:53	0:19:25	0:38:50	1:21:55	2:43:49
0:03:54	0:19:30	0:39:00	1:22:16	2:44:32
0:03:55	0:19:35	0:39:10	1:22:37	2:45:14
0:03:56	0:19:40	0:39:20	1:22:58	2:45:56
0:03:57	0:19:45	0:39:30	1:23:19	2:46:38
0:03:58	0:19:50	0:39:40	1:23:40	2:47:20
0:03:59	0:19:55	0:39:50	1:24:01	2:48:02
0:04:00	0:20:00	0:40:00	1:24:22	2:48:45
0:04:01	0:20:05	0:40:10	1:24:43	2:49:27
0:04:02	0:20:10	0:40:20	1:25:05	2:50:09
0:04:03	0:20:15	0:40:30	1:25:26	2:50:51
0:04:04	0:20:20	0:40:40	1:25:47	2:51:33
0:04:05	0:20:25	0:40:50	1:26:08	2:52:16
0:04:06	0:20:30	0:41:00	1:26:29	2:52:58
0:04:07	0:20:35	0:41:10	1:26:50	2:53:40
0:04:08	0:20:40	0:41:20	1:27:11	2:54:22
0:04:09	0:20:45	0:41:30	1:27:32	2:55:04
0:04:10	0:20:50	0:41:40	1:27:53	2:55:46
0:04:11	0:20:55	0:41:50	1:28:14	2:56:29
0:04:12	0:21:00	0:42:00	1:28:35	2:57:11
0:04:13	0:21:05	0:42:10	1:28:57	2:57:53
0:04:14	0:21:10	0:42:20	1:29:18	2:58:35
0:04:15	0:21:15	0:42:30	1:29:39	2:59:17
0:04:16	0:21:20	0:42:40	1:30:00	3:00:00
0:04:17	0:21:25	0:42:50	1:30:21	3:00:42
0:04:18	0:21:30	0:43:00	1:30:42	3:01:24
0:04:19	0:21:35	0:43:10	1:31:03	3:02:06
0:04:20	0:21:40	0:43:20	1:31:24	3:02:48
0:04:21	0:21:45	0:43:30	1:31:45	3:03:31
0:04:22	0:21:50	0:43:40	1:32:06	3:04:13

MM:SS/KM	5K	10K	HALF-MARATHON	MARATHON
0:04:23	0:21:55	0:43:50	1:32:27	3:04:55
0:04:24	0:22:00	0:44:00	1:32:49	3:05:37
0:04:25	0:22:05	0:44:10	1:33:10	3:06:19
0:04:26	0:22:10	0:44:20	1:33:31	3:07:01
0:04:27	0:22:15	0:44:30	1:33:52	3:07:44
0:04:28	0:22:20	0:44:40	1:34:13	3:08:26
0:04:29	0:22:25	0:44:50	1:34:34	3:09:08
0:04:30	0:22:30	0:45:00	1:34:55	3:09:50
0:04:31	0:22:35	0:45:10	1:35:16	3:10:32
0:04:32	0:22:40	0:45:20	1:35:37	3:11:15
0:04:33	0:22:45	0:45:30	1:35:58	3:11:57
0:04:34	0:22:50	0:45:40	1:36:19	3:12:39
0:04:35	0:22:55	0:45:50	1:36:41	3:13:21
0:04:36	0:23:00	0:46:00	1:37:02	3:14:03
0:04:37	0:23:05	0:46:10	1:37:23	3:14:46
0:04:38	0:23:10	0:46:20	1:37:44	3:15:28
0:04:39	0:23:15	0:46:30	1:38:05	3:16:10
0:04:40	0:23:20	0:46:40	1:38:26	3:16:52
0:04:41	0:23:25	0:46:50	1:38:47	3:17:34
0:04:42	0:23:30	0:47:00	1:39:08	3:18:16
0:04:43	0:23:35	0:47:10	1:39:29	3:18:59
0:04:44	0:23:40	0:47:20	1:39:50	3:19:41
0:04:45	0:23:45	0:47:30	1:40:12	3:20:23
0:04:46	0:23:50	0:47:40	1:40:33	3:21:05
0:04:47	0:23:55	0:47:50	1:40:54	3:21:47
0:04:48	0:24:00	0:48:00	1:41:15	3:22:30
0:04:49	0:24:05	0:48:10	1:41:36	3:23:12
0:04:50	0:24:10	0:48:20	1:41:57	3:23:54
0:04:51	0:24:15	0:48:30	1:42:18	3:24:36
0:04:52	0:24:20	0:48:40	1:42:39	3:25:18
0:04:53	0:24:25	0:48:50	1:43:00	3:26:00
0:04:54	0:24:30	0:49:00	1:43:21	3:26:43
0:04:55	0:24:35	0:49:10	1:43:42	3:27:25
0:04:56	0:24:40	0:49:20	1:44:04	3:28:07
0:04:57	0:24:45	0:49:30	1:44:25	3:28:49
0:04:58	0:24:50	0:49:40	1:44:46	3:29:31
0:04:59	0:24:55	0:49:50	1:45:07	3:30:14
0:05:00	0:25:00	0:50:00	1:45:28	3:30:56
0:05:01	0:25:05	0:50:10	1:45:49	3:31:38
0:05:02	0:25:10	0:50:20	1:46:10	3:32:20

MM:SS/KM	5K	10K	HALF-MARATHON	MARATHON
0:05:03	0:25:15	0:50:30	1:46:31	3:33:02
0:05:04	0:25:20	0:50:40	1:46:52	3:33:45
0:05:05	0:25:25	0:50:50	1:47:13	3:34:27
0:05:06	0:25:30	0:51:00	1:47:34	3:35:09
0:05:07	0:25:35	0:51:10	1:47:56	3:35:51
0:05:08	0:25:40	0:51:20	1:48:17	3:36:33
0:05:09	0:25:45	0:51:30	1:48:38	3:37:15
0:05:10	0:25:50	0:51:40	1:48:59	3:37:58
0:05:11	0:25:55	0:51:50	1:49:20	3:38:40
0:05:12	0:26:00	0:52:00	1:49:41	3:39:22
0:05:13	0:26:05	0:52:10	1:50:02	3:40:04
0:05:14	0:26:10	0:52:20	1:50:23	3:40:46
0:05:15	0:26:15	0:52:30	1:50:44	3:41:29
0:05:16	0:26:20	0:52:40	1:51:05	3:42:11
0:05:17	0:26:25	0:52:50	1:51:26	3:42:53
0:05:18	0:26:30	0:53:00	1:51:48	3:43:35
0:05:19	0:26:35	0:53:10	1:52:09	3:44:17
0:05:20	0:26:40	0:53:20	1:52:30	3:45:00
0:05:21	0:26:45	0:53:30	1:52:51	3:45:42
0:05:22	0:26:50	0:53:40	1:53:12	3:46:24
0:05:23	0:26:55	0:53:50	1:53:33	3:47:06
0:05:24	0:27:00	0:54:00	1:53:54	3:47:48
0:05:25	0:27:05	0:54:10	1:54:15	3:48:30
0:05:26	0:27:10	0:54:20	1:54:36	3:49:13
0:05:27	0:27:15	0:54:30	1:54:57	3:49:55
0:05:28	0:27:20	0:54:40	1:55:19	3:50:37
0:05:29	0:27:25	0:54:50	1:55:40	3:51:19
0:05:30	0:27:30	0:55:00	1:56:01	3:52:01
0:05:31	0:27:35	0:55:10	1:56:22	3:52:44
0:05:32	0:27:40	0:55:20	1:56:43	3:53:26
0:05:33	0:27:45	0:55:30	1:57:04	3:54:08
0:05:34	0:27:50	0:55:40	1:57:25	3:54:50
0:05:35	0:27:55	0:55:50	1:57:46	3:55:32
0:05:36	0:28:00	0:56:00	1:58:07	3:56:14
0:05:37	0:28:05	0:56:10	1:58:28	3:56:57
0:05:38	0:28:10	0:56:20	1:58:49	3:57:39
0:05:39	0:28:15	0:56:30	1:59:11	3:58:21
0:05:40	0:28:20	0:56:40	1:59:32	3:59:03
0:05:41	0:28:25	0:56:50	1:59:53	3:59:45
0:05:42	0:28:30	0:57:00	2:00:14	4:00:28

MM:SS/KM	5K	10K	HALF-MARATHON	MARATHON
0:05:43	0:28:35	0:57:10	2:00:35	4:01:10
0:05:44	0:28:40	0:57:20	2:00:56	4:01:52
0:05:45	0:28:45	0:57:30	2:01:17	4:02:34
0:05:46	0:28:50	0:57:40	2:01:38	4:03:16
0:05:47	0:28:55	0:57:50	2:01:59	4:03:59
0:05:48	0:29:00	0:58:00	2:02:20	4:04:41
0:05:49	0:29:05	0:58:10	2:02:41	4:05:23
0:05:50	0:29:10	0:58:20	2:03:03	4:06:05
0:05:51	0:29:15	0:58:30	2:03:24	4:06:47
0:05:52	0:29:20	0:58:40	2:03:45	4:07:29
0:05:53	0:29:25	0:58:50	2:04:06	4:08:12
0:05:54	0:29:30	0:59:00	2:04:27	4:08:54
0:05:55	0:29:35	0:59:10	2:04:48	4:09:36
0:05:56	0:29:40	0:59:20	2:05:09	4:10:18
0:05:57	0:29:45	0:59:30	2:05:30	4:11:00
0:05:58	0:29:50	0:59:40	2:05:51	4:11:43
0:05:59	0:29:55	0:59:50	2:06:12	4:12:25
0:06:00	0:30:00	1:00:00	2:06:33	4:13:07
0:06:01	0:30:05	1:00:10	2:06:55	4:13:49
0:06:02	0:30:10	1:00:20	2:07:16	4:14:31
0:06:03	0:30:15	1:00:30	2:07:37	4:15:14
0:06:04	0:30:20	1:00:40	2:07:58	4:15:56
0:06:05	0:30:25	1:00:50	2:08:19	4:16:38
0:06:06	0:30:30	1:01:00	2:08:40	4:17:20
0:06:07	0:30:35	1:01:10	2:09:01	4:18:02
0:06:08	0:30:40	1:01:20	2:09:22	4:18:44
0:06:09	0:30:45	1:01:30	2:09:43	4:19:27
0:06:10	0:30:50	1:01:40	2:10:04	4:20:09
0:06:11	0:30:55	1:01:50	2:10:26	4:20:51
0:06:12	0:31:00	1:02:00	2:10:47	4:21:33
0:06:13	0:31:05	1:02:10	2:11:08	4:22:15
0:06:14	0:31:10	1:02:20	2:11:29	4:22:58
0:06:15	0:31:15	1:02:30	2:11:50	4:23:40
0:06:16	0:31:20	1:02:40	2:12:11	4:24:22
0:06:17	0:31:25	1:02:50	2:12:32	4:25:04
0:06:18	0:31:30	1:03:00	2:12:53	4:25:46
0:06:19	0:31:35	1:03:10	2:13:14	4:26:28
0:06:20	0:31:40	1:03:20	2:13:35	4:27:11
0:06:21	0:31:45	1:03:30	2:13:56	4:27:53
0:06:22	0:31:50	1:03:40	2:14:18	4:28:35

MM:SS/KM	5K	10K	HALF-MARATHON	MARATHON
0:06:23	0:31:55	1:03:50	2:14:39	4:29:17
0:06:24	0:32:00	1:04:00	2:15:00	4:29:59
0:06:25	0:32:05	1:04:10	2:15:21	4:30:42
0:06:26	0:32:10	1:04:20	2:15:42	4:31:24
0:06:27	0:32:15	1:04:30	2:16:03	4:32:06
0:06:28	0:32:20	1:04:40	2:16:24	4:32:48
0:06:29	0:32:25	1:04:50	2:16:45	4:33:30
0:06:30	0:32:30	1:05:00	2:17:06	4:34:13
0:06:31	0:32:35	1:05:10	2:17:27	4:34:55
0:06:32	0:32:40	1:05:20	2:17:48	4:35:37
0:06:33	0:32:45	1:05:30	2:18:10	4:36:19
0:06:34	0:32:50	1:05:40	2:18:31	4:37:01
0:06:35	0:32:55	1:05:50	2:18:52	4:37:43
0:06:36	0:33:00	1:06:00	2:19:13	4:38:26
0:06:37	0:33:05	1:06:10	2:19:34	4:39:08
0:06:38	0:33:10	1:06:20	2:19:55	4:39:50
0:06:39	0:33:15	1:06:30	2:20:16	4:40:32
0:06:40	0:33:20	1:06:40	2:20:37	4:41:14
0:06:41	0:33:25	1:06:50	2:20:58	4:41:57
0:06:42	0:33:30	1:07:00	2:21:19	4:42:39
0:06:43	0:33:35	1:07:10	2:21:40	4:43:21
0:06:44	0:33:40	1:07:20	2:22:02	4:44:03
0:06:45	0:33:45	1:07:30	2:22:23	4:44:45
0:06:46	0:33:50	1:07:40	2:22:44	4:45:28
0:06:47	0:33:55	1:07:50	2:23:05	4:46:10
0:06:48	0:34:00	1:08:00	2:23:26	4:46:52
0:06:49	0:34:05	1:08:10	2:23:47	4:47:34
0:06:50	0:34:10	1:08:20	2:24:08	4:48:16
0:06:51	0:34:15	1:08:30	2:24:29	4:48:58
0:06:52	0:34:20	1:08:40	2:24:50	4:49:41
0:06:53	0:34:25	1:08:50	2:25:11	4:50:23
0:06:54	0:34:30	1:09:00	2:25:33	4:51:05
0:06:55	0:34:35	1:09:10	2:25:54	4:51:47
0:06:56	0:34:40	1:09:20	2:26:15	4:52:29
0:06:57	0:34:45	1:09:30	2:26:36	4:53:12
0:06:58	0:34:50	1:09:40	2:26:57	4:53:54
0:06:59	0:34:55	1:09:50	2:27:18	4:54:36
0:07:00	0:35:00	1:10:00	2:27:39	4:55:18
0:07:01	0:35:05	1:10:10	2:28:00	4:56:00
0:07:02	0:35:10	1:10:20	2:28:21	4:56:43

MM:SS/KM	5K	10K	HALF-MARATHON	MARATHON
0:07:03	0:35:15	1:10:30	2:28:42	4:57:25
0:07:04	0:35:20	1:10:40	2:29:03	4:58:07
0:07:05	0:35:25	1:10:50	2:29:25	4:58:49
0:07:06	0:35:30	1:11:00	2:29:46	4:59:31
0:07:07	0:35:35	1:11:10	2:30:07	5:00:13
0:07:08	0:35:40	1:11:20	2:30:28	5:00:56
0:07:09	0:35:45	1:11:30	2:30:49	5:01:38
0:07:10	0:35:50	1:11:40	2:31:10	5:02:20
0:07:11	0:35:55	1:11:50	2:31:31	5:03:02
0:07:12	0:36:00	1:12:00	2:31:52	5:03:44
0:07:13	0:36:05	1:12:10	2:32:13	5:04:27
0:07:14	0:36:10	1:12:20	2:32:34	5:05:09
0:07:15	0:36:15	1:12:30	2:32:55	5:05:51
0:07:16	0:36:20	1:12:40	2:33:17	5:06:33
0:07:17	0:36:25	1:12:50	2:33:38	5:07:15
0:07:18	0:36:30	1:13:00	2:33:59	5:07:57
0:07:19	0:36:35	1:13:10	2:34:20	5:08:40
0:07:20	0:36:40	1:13:20	2:34:41	5:09:22
0:07:21	0:36:45	1:13:30	2:35:02	5:10:04
0:07:22	0:36:50	1:13:40	2:35:23	5:10:46
0:07:23	0:36:55	1:13:50	2:35:44	5:11:28
0:07:24	0:37:00	1:14:00	2:36:05	5:12:11
0:07:25	0:37:05	1:14:10	2:36:26	5:12:53
0:07:26	0:37:10	1:14:20	2:36:47	5:13:35
0:07:27	0:37:15	1:14:30	2:37:09	5:14:17
0:07:28	0:37:20	1:14:40	2:37:30	5:14:59
0:07:29	0:37:25	1:14:50	2:37:51	5:15:42
0:07:30	0:37:30	1:15:00	2:38:12	5:16:24
0:07:31	0:37:35	1:15:10	2:38:33	5:17:06
0:07:32	0:37:40	1:15:20	2:38:54	5:17:48
0:07:33	0:37:45	1:15:30	2:39:15	5:18:30
0:07:34	0:37:50	1:15:40	2:39:36	5:19:12
0:07:35	0:37:55	1:15:50	2:39:57	5:19:55
0:07:36	0:38:00	1:16:00	2:40:18	5:20:37
0:07:37	0:38:05	1:16:10	2:40:40	5:21:19
0:07:38	0:38:10	1:16:20	2:41:01	5:22:01
0:07:39	0:38:15	1:16:30	2:41:22	5:22:43
0:07:40	0:38:20	1:16:40	2:41:43	5:23:26
0:07:41	0:38:25	1:16:50	2:42:04	5:24:08
0:07:42	0:38:30	1:17:00	2:42:25	5:24:50

MM:SS/KM	5K	10K	HALF-MARATHON	MARATHON
0:07:43	0:38:35	1:17:10	2:42:46	5:25:32
0:07:44	0:38:40	1:17:20	2:43:07	5:26:14
0:07:45	0:38:45	1:17:30	2:43:28	5:26:56
0:07:46	0:38:50	1:17:40	2:43:49	5:27:39
0:07:47	0:38:55	1:17:50	2:44:10	5:28:21
0:07:48	0:39:00	1:18:00	2:44:32	5:29:03
0:07:49	0:39:05	1:18:10	2:44:53	5:29:45
0:07:50	0:39:10	1:18:20	2:45:14	5:30:27
0:07:51	0:39:15	1:18:30	2:45:35	5:31:10
0:07:52	0:39:20	1:18:40	2:45:56	5:31:52
0:07:53	0:39:25	1:18:50	2:46:17	5:32:34
0:07:54	0:39:30	1:19:00	2:46:38	5:33:16
0:07:55	0:39:35	1:19:10	2:46:59	5:33:58
0:07:56	0:39:40	1:19:20	2:47:20	5:34:41
0:07:57	0:39:45	1:19:30	2:47:41	5:35:23
0:07:58	0:39:50	1:19:40	2:48:02	5:36:05
0:07:59	0:39:55	1:19:50	2:48:24	5:36:47
0:08:00	0:40:00	1:20:00	2:48:45	5:37:29
0:08:01	0:40:05	1:20:10	2:49:06	5:38:11
0:08:02	0:40:10	1:20:20	2:49:27	5:38:54
0:08:03	0:40:15	1:20:30	2:49:48	5:39:36

INDEX

Underscored page references indicate charts and tables.

A